Surgical Consent

SURGICAL CONSENT
Bioethics and Cochlear Implantation

Linda Komesaroff
Editor

Gallaudet University Press
Washington, D.C.

Washington, DC 20002
http://gupress.gallaudet.edu

© 2007 by Gallaudet University
All rights reserved. Published 2007
Printed in the United States of America

Library of Congress Cataloging-in-Publication Data

Surgical consent : bioethics and cochlear implantation / Linda Komesaroff, editor.
    p. ; cm.
Includes bibliographical references and index.
ISBN 978-1-56368-349-7 (alk. paper)
    1. Cochlear implants—Moral and ethical aspects.   2. Deaf—Rehabilitation—Moral
and ethical aspects.   3. Deaf children—Rehabilitation—Moral and ethical aspects.
I. Komesaroff, Linda R.
    [DNLM: 1. Cochlear Implantation—ethics.   2. Cochlear Implantation—psychology.
3. Deafness—psychology.   4. Deafness—surgery.   5. Disabled Children—psychology.
6. Hearing Impaired Persons—psychology.   7. Parental Consent—ethics. WV 274 S961 2007]
    RF305.S85 2007
    174'.96178822—dc22
                                                                2007007004

♾ The paper used in this publication meets the minimum requirements for American
National Standard for Information Sciences—Permanence of Paper for Printed Library
Materials, ANSI Z39.48-1984.

CONTENTS

FOREWORD

This work is an edited volume by Deaf and hearing authors about issues of bio-ethics and deaf people. It brings together diverse perspectives on cochlear implantation in a series of essays from ethicists, educators, and Deaf leaders. The contributing authors were asked to respond to the issue of childhood implantation in relation to their discipline and a number of themes of enquiry: human rights, medical and social ethics, psychology, education, globalization, identity, life pathways, democracy, media, law, and biotechnology. Drawing on current research, they provide insight into the different responses to the high rate of implantation around the globe. Their chapters provide alternate views to the medicalized perspective of deafness overwhelmingly communicated through the media and those who work in the cochlear implantation industry. This work was also an opportunity to foreground the views of Deaf experts, their voices articulate and, at times, raw.

The book is characterized by the use of social critical theories by a number of authors who seek to understand the relationships between deaf people and the dominant hearing society in which they live. It relocates what is traditionally seen as a medical issue within social, cultural, and political domains. At the same time, it attempts to disrupt the dichotomies that have long dominated the field of deafness—speech versus sign, instruction through speech and sign systems versus bilingual education, and medical intervention versus cultural membership to the Deaf community.

This volume was originally conceived with the help of Markku Jokinen, Deaf academic and president of the World Federation of the Deaf. His encouragement and contacts were invaluable, and his support for the importance of this publication is very much appreciated.

Linda Komesaroff
Editor

CONTRIBUTORS

Priscilla Alderson is a professor in the faculty of education at the University of London, London, U.K.

Inger Lise Skog Hansen is a researcher at the Fafo Institute for Labour and Social Research, Oslo, Norway.

Hilde Haualand is a social anthropologist at the Fafo Institute for Labour and Social Research, Oslo, Norway.

Linda Komesaroff is a senior lecturer in the faculty of education at Deakin University, Melbourne, Australia.

Paddy Ladd is a senior lecturer and Deaf activist at the Centre for Deaf Studies at the University of Bristol, Bristol, U.K.

Harlan Lane is a professor of psychology and linguistics at Northeastern University, Boston, Massachusetts, U.S.

Karen Lloyd is a Deaf leader and manager of the Australian Association of the Deaf.

Eithne Mills is a senior lecturer in the School of Law at Deakin University, Melbourne, Australia.

Paal Richard Peterson is a Deaf political scientist from Oslo, Norway.

Gunilla Preisler is a professor in the Department of Psychology at Stockholm University, Stockholm, Sweden.

Kristina Svartholm is a professor in the Department of Scandinavian Languages at Stockholm University, Stockholm, Sweden.

Michael Uniacke is a Deaf author and freelance writer from Melbourne, Australia.

INTRODUCTION

This current time is a critical moment in the field of deafness internationally. More than twenty years since the first cochlear implant system gained clearance for use by adults in the United States, the cochlear implant has become the dominant approach to treating congenital deafness among people in most Western countries. In 1987, approximately 500 people throughout the world had cochlear implants (Slee 1987); by the following year, more than 3,000 people had been implanted (Randal 1988, 11). The first cochlear implant system for use by children (from the age of two years) gained clearance in 1990 from the Food and Drug Administration in the United States; the minimum age for implantation dropped to eighteen months in 1998 and to twelve months the following year. Babies as young as five months are now being implanted. As the age at implantation has dropped, the number of implant recipients has continued to soar.

In 1990, an estimated 5,000 people had implants worldwide (Christiansen and Leigh 2002). In 1997, the figure rose to 16,000; by 2002, it was almost 60,000; and according to 2005 data, there are nearly 100,000 implant recipients (National Institute on Deafness and other Communication Disorders 2002, 2006). Christiansen and Leigh (2002) add a caveat to implantation statistics: the number of users is less than the number of recipients, although this number is unknown.

Cochlear, the leading manufacturer of cochlear implants in the world, reportedly accounts for 70 percent of the global cochlear implant market—and considers that percentage as only 10 percent of the potential market (Cochlear 2005). Its chief executive officer, Chris Roberts, predicts that bilateral implantation (the implantation of devices in both ears) could be routine within the decade, telling *Business Week Online* that "current implant patients could end up being excellent repeat customers" (Einhorn 2005). The company currently sells its products to more than seventy countries and continues to expand its export base into the United States, Asia Pacific, Europe, and the Middle East through an aggressive program of global penetration. In many regions, implantation is made possible through sponsored medical programs that are financed by governments or charitable donations.

The recent announcement of an inquiry by the U.S. Department of Justice into Cochlear America's relationships with healthcare professionals again plunged this industry into the headlines. The economic implication of such a move dominated the business pages of the national and international press, as did an earlier report of deaths from meningitis linked to U.S. implants (see Komesaroff, this volume). The result was a drop in the share price and reported downturn in Cochlear's sales across Europe. It was not long, however, before the market recovered and the manufacturer again reported all-time records in the company's profitability and return to shareholders (Cochlear 2005). Economic imperatives—such as the global market place, the commercialization of medical intervention, and the effect of negative publicity—are critical to the discussion of cochlear implantation.

The rate of childhood implantation in many countries is now estimated to involve 90 percent–95 percent of all children born deaf. The number of children implanted since 1990 has increased from one in ten total recipients to one in two recipients in 2002 (Christiansen and Leigh 2002). The implementation of programs to screen the hearing of newborns, including programs recently introduced in the United States and Australia, has resulted in children being identified and referred to implant clinics at a very young age. The Sydney Cochlear Implant Clinic (SCIC), for example, reports that 93 percent of profoundly deaf children in New South Wales are now being referred to it for assessment (SCIC n.d.). With the high rate of childhood implantation worldwide, the historical split between spoken and signed languages is poised to become even deeper. At the same time, the emerging field of gene technology continues to push the debate about the nature of deafness, medical intervention, and the future of Deaf communities beyond the question of cochlear implantation. The contributors to this volume have considered cochlear implants within this broader field of biotechnology.

This volume starts and ends with the voices of Deaf people. Their essays provide a penetrating view into the concerns of Deaf leaders, academics, and researchers who, in my view, have the strongest speaking rights about issues that affect Deaf people. At the same time, their insight into issues of power, positioning, and minority–majority group relations are critical to the dominant group's understanding of diversity and globalization.

The use of capitalized *Deaf* generally distinguishes those people who are deaf (in the medical sense of the word) and who use sign language and consider themselves to be part of the Deaf community, a cultural and linguistic minority. Where the cultural and linguistic status of deaf individuals is unknown or diverse, most authors have used the term *deaf;* making reference to deaf children, deaf education, and teachers of the deaf. A stronger view is held by academic and Deaf rights activist, Paddy Ladd. In the opening chapter, Ladd uses *Deaf* for all contexts— referring to Deaf children, teachers of the Deaf and Deaf education. Deaf children, in his view, are automatically members of "Sign Language Peoples" (a term he coins to identify the importance of sign language to these people) and thus, to Deaf communities. His use of the latter terms—teachers of the Deaf, and *Deaf education*—adopt the capitalized *Deaf* in a bid to reclaim their education and decolonize the territory of Sign Language Peoples. In a similar vein, his reference to *Oralism* is capitalized as a marker of the colonialist tradition forced onto Deaf peoples. Despite differences between Ladd and other authors in the degree to which the politicalization of deafness is highlighted, his chapter in this volume provides the context for later chapters. It unpacks the ways in which Deafness has been constructed by the dominant society and situates cochlear implants within broader social contexts. Ladd presents a powerful and highly theorized account of colonialism (and the waves of neocolonialism) that frames the topic of cochlear implantation. Cochlear implantation, he says, is just the latest in a number of waves of neocolonialism that have swept over Deaf people and their rights. His historical account of the response to cochlear implantation by deafness organizations in the United Kingdom provides the reader with an inside view of the struggle for human rights and response to biotechnology. He warns that the possibility that signed language training is "added" for implant recipients is a rationalized approach by those who believe that although cochlear implantation cannot be halted it nonetheless results in a breach of deaf children's rights.

In chapter 2, Harlan Lane, professor at Northeastern University in Boston, Massachusetts, develops a robust argument for the recognition of Deaf ethnicity and the Deaf world. He deconstructs (and debunks) the medicalized view of deaf people as members of a disability group. Predicated on a misunderstanding, the disability construction of deafness, he says, brings "bad solutions to real problems."

In chapter 3, Linda Komesaroff, a senior lecturer at Deakin University, Melbourne, presents a comprehensive analysis of the media representation of cochlear implants from articles that appeared in the daily press in the first decade of media exposure. Her analysis identifies the ways in which the press has characterized deafness and biotechnology as well as the ways that members of the dominant group have positioned deaf people within society. A textual analysis of a sample of articles highlights the devices used by authors (deaf and hearing) to represent their world views and to position the reader in the debate.

Chapters 4 and 5 deal with issues of medical ethics and legal rights. In chapter 4, Priscilla Alderson, professor from the University of London, reviews the background social and ethical debates and decision-making frameworks concerned with surgery for children. She views cochlear implants as part of the powerful social trend to use technical aids to alter, adapt, or "improve" the natural body. She takes a critical social perspective of cochlear implantation, highlighting the importance of informed decision making, critical thinking, and choice making (avoiding assumptions and trends that may otherwise be taken for granted). She asks: "Whom do they really benefit? Are such aids as essential and beneficial as is usually claimed?" If people do little reflection on such questions, she suggests that people are then liable to opt for the treatment in question, believing "TINA—There Is No Alternative."

Chapter 5 is written by lawyer Eithne Mills, from Deakin University, Melbourne. Beginning with the United Nations *Declaration of the Rights of the Child*, she considers the interaction between medicine and the law in cases related to medical intervention. She introduces the reader to key legal doctrines, international conventions, and established general precedents that must be understood in relation to legal action and medical intervention such as implantation in childhood. The chapter begins with a discussion of patriarchal power, the rights of the child, and the principle of "best interests" in family law. The second part of the chapter discusses what constitutes *valid consent* and analyzes three cases of medical intervention in children. The third case was heard in the Federal Magistrates Court of Australia in relation to a dispute between two deaf parents involving issues of residence and contact as well as disagreement over the implantation of their profoundly deaf child who was age eighteen months. The child's mother had applied to the court seeking authorization of the proposed medical intervention involving the implantation of a cochlear device. The court noted that at the heart of the dispute were the parents' differing views about how their deaf child should be raised in a mainly hearing world.

Chapters 6, 7, and 8 relate to deaf children's psychological, social, and educational development. Chapter 6 by Gunilla Preisler, a professor at Stockholm University, Sweden, reports the analysis and results of a study of the psychosocial development of deaf children with cochlear implants in Sweden. Her colleague at Stockholm University, Kristina Svartholm (chapter 7), considers the ways in which children with cochlear implants can be accommodated in Sweden's bilingual schools and the implications for the school system. In Chapter 8, Hilde

Haualand and Inger Hansen, social science researchers at the Fafo Institute in Oslo, present the results of their study of communication among Norwegian deaf and hard of hearing children. Their findings challenge the assumption made by cochlear implant supporters that being hearing impaired is "better than" being deaf.

The final two chapters in this volume are written by Deaf contributors. In chapter 9, Norwegian Deaf political scientist, Paal Richard Peterson, questions how Deaf people's freedom of speech can be secured given that cochlear implants do not provide recipients with perfect hearing. He asks whether cochlear implant recipients who are not supported in using their native signed language can be said to be active participants in a democratic society. He provides very interesting examples of Deaf people's political participation as well as the things that are needed for respectful communication and equal access to information. The final chapter (chapter 10) is written by two Deaf Australians, Karen Lloyd, manager of the Australian Association of the Deaf, and Michael Uniacke, an Australian deaf journalist and freelance writer. Their report "from ground level," as they call it, presents their accumulated sixty years of experience mixing with other deaf and hard of hearing people. Their voices are strong and, at times, impassioned as they provide an honest account of their backgrounds, views, and concerns. This highly personalized chapter provides a fascinating insight into the beliefs of two Deaf adults who move in the heart of the Deaf community.

REFERENCES

Christiansen, J. B., and I. W. Leigh. 2002. *Cochlear implants in children: Ethics and choices*. Washington D.C.: Gallaudet University Press.

Cochlear. 2005. Annual Report 2005. http://www.cochlear.com/Corp/Investor/AnnualReport2005/intro.htm

Einhorn, B., with Symonds, W. C. 2005. Listen: The sound of hope—cochlear implants could be a boon for the deaf . . . and a booming business. *Business Week Online*, November 14. http://www.businessweek.com/magazine/content/05_46/b3959101.htm.

National Institute of Health. 1995. Cochlear implants in adults and children. *NIH Consensus Statement Online*, 13 (2, May 15–17):1–30. http://www.medhelp.org/lib/100coc.htm.

National Institute on Deafness and Other Communication Disorders. 2002. Cochlear implants (fact sheet). http://www.nidcd.nih.gov/health/hearing/coch.htm.

National Institute on Deafness and Other Communication Disorders. 2006. Cochlear implants (fact sheet). http://www.nidcd.nih.gov/health/hearing/coch.htm.

Randal, J. E. 1988. Your health: Implants for the hearing-impaired. *Newsday*, May 24, 11.

Slee, A. 1987. Lack of funds threatens bionic ear development. *Sydney Morning Herald*, August 8, 13.

Sydney Cochlear Implant Centre (SCIC). n.d. Outcomes. http://www.scic.nsw.gov.au/showarticle.asp?faq=2&fldAuto=52&header=header2.

1

COCHLEAR IMPLANTATION, COLONIALISM, AND DEAF RIGHTS

Paddy Ladd

This chapter examines the issue of childhood cochlear implantation against the background of the situation for Deaf people in the United Kingdom (with reference to other countries where relevant). It is my belief that one reason for the lack of success in critiquing or challenging cochlear implantation is that Deaf discourses in general, and Deaf studies in particular, have been overwhelmingly inwardly focused; Deaf issues are discussed almost in intellectual isolation from the wider political patterns of world events. Thus, this chapter takes pains to extend the frame of reference for discussion of this issue. In particular, the concept of colonialism,[1] as it pertains to signed language communities, is used to frame and evaluate issues related to cochlear implantation. I also introduce a new concept of "positive" and "negative" biology as a bridge to similar emergent concepts in other disciplines such as women's studies. Wrigley (1996) concisely frames the issue:

> What new colony in the name of communications technology is sited on the body of the Deaf? What discovery by a new "Columbus" is re-enacted on this new "continent" of language and communication? Did anyone notice any natives? (206)

COLONIALISM AND SIGN LANGUAGE PEOPLES

The discourses of sign language peoples (SLPs), as I term them, and those who have administered those communities have been diametrically opposed for the past 120 (or more) years. At the root of their difference are the conceptualizations of deafness and Deaf people. The primary difference has been one of perception. Deaf people often see themselves as linguistically and culturally complete human beings. Moreover, during the SLPs' more self-confident eras, their epistemologies and ontologies have stressed what I have termed "positive biology" (Ladd and West, forthcoming); that is, through their biological differences, SLPs

My thanks go to the following people (and those who could not be named) for their help with aspects of this chapter: Kay Alexander, Jen Dodds, Mike Gulliver, Claire Haddon, Linda Komesaroff, Harlan Lane, Raymond Lee, Karen Page, and Joe Santini.

have developed skills and faculties that are underused and thus underappreciated by hearing-speaking populations.

Features of Deaf people's positive biology include enhanced visual skills; sensitivity to touch and enhanced general tactility; and enhanced use of face, hands, and bodies. Indeed, Deaf languages have emerged from precisely this foundation. These qualities have led to a remarkably high degree of globalism among Deaf people; the syntactic similarities and profound "plasticity" of their languages has led to their belief that SLPs set a contrasting example to the (hearing) human history of war and oppression. This positive example of human diversity is a gift that SLPs offer to the rest of the human race (compare Mottez 1993) and is a significant contribution to what constitutes human knowledge. This perspective is perhaps best encapsulated by the expression used by the great American Deaf leader, George Veditz, in his description of Deaf peoples as "Peoples of the Eye" (see Crouch 1941/1998).

By contrast, negative biology, the hegemonic professional discourse used in the field of deafness, is the perception of SLPs as medically deficient and in need of a cure. The problem created for Deaf communities lies in the imbalance in power between Deaf and hearing people that results from this discourse. Following Lane (1993) and Wrigley (1996), I have argued elsewhere that it is not possible to effect a shift in the balance of power without a sophisticated understanding of how it has come to be constructed and how it manifests itself in Deaf people's lives (Ladd 2003). I submit that the model of colonialism is one step toward such understanding. Colonialism is best understood here as linguistic, cultural, and social-welfare colonization, although Lane suggests that economic colonization is also present.

Once we step into the domains of postcolonialist discourse, we are able to identify parallels between SLPs and other colonized peoples. Moreover, we note that considerable differences exist in how the various forms of colonialism manifest themselves on each of those peoples. Each have their own particular bete noires, whether they be missionaries, mining companies, military contractors or social workers, even including Native Americans' especial anger toward anthropologists (Deloria 1988). These differences are important, not least of all because the thrust of audist colonialism comes from what conventional postcolonialist theory might perceive to be an atypical colonialist domain—the biomedical domain. However, the focus on biological dimensions is also found in the treatment of other colonized peoples such as nineteenth-century medical attempts to prove Black inferiority through measurement of skull sizes or twentieth-century psychology that pathologized cultural differences (compare Lane 1993).

It is important to note the dynamics of how SLPs have been administered by colonizing forces. Certain members of administrative professions (doctors, audiologists, teachers, and so on) have been selected and entrusted to undertake this work on behalf, and in the name, of the wider lay population. Interestingly, the attitudes of lay people toward Deaf people may well have been more positive than the attitudes of those who have carried out the colonialization of peoples who use sign languages, supposedly on their behalf. Therefore, the control of information to the wider society is a key aspect of this form of colonialism; the control of media discourses is something that colonizing forces give high priority. The professionals in question are located in education, with reinforcement from those in the medical and technological professions. With respect to Deaf adults, these groups are augmented by charitable organizations and social welfare professions; in both cases, as normally occurs in hegemonic discourses, the members of these professions maintain a virtually exclusive relationship with government politicians and administrators.

At various times in history, Deaf people and their allies have been able to penetrate this discursive system, achieving some amelioration of oppressive policies and, at times, have even taken significant steps toward decolonization (for a description of the successful Deaf President Now protest at Gallaudet University, Washington, D.C., in 1988, see Malzkuhn, Covell, Hlibok, and Bourne-Firl 1994; Jankowski 1997; Christiansen and Barnartt 2002).

However, in the wider world, so-called decolonization has turned out to be a chimera. Underlying structures of traditional colonialism are perpetuated, for example, by Western economies, the International Monetary Fund, and the World Bank through economic control of former colonies—sustaining forms that have become known as neocolonialism. Unlike earlier forms of colonization, these newer forms are characterized by being carried out at a distance and, thus, by a lack of visibility. In a similar manner, three distinct waves of neocolonialism have recently been enacted on Deaf populations: mainstreaming, cochlear implant experimentation, and genetic modification.

Neocolonialism and Sign Language Peoples

The removal of "the Deaf variety" of the human race has appeared before as a goal of colonialism (see Lane, 1984). The latest three waves of neocolonialism, however, have even more explicitly been intended to destroy the existence of Deaf communities, isolating Deaf children from one another so that opportunities for Deaf enculturation are minimized. These three waves of neocolonialism—mainstreaming, cochlear implant experimentation, and genetic modification—are interconnected, and although the topic of this chapter is primarily concerned with the second of these attempts at colonialism, it is crucial to our understanding of cochlear implantation that it cannot be properly analyzed without reference to its relationship with the other two.

These three waves of neocolonialism differ significantly from older forms of colonialism of SLPs. First, the discourse of mainstreaming has gained consent from (and, indeed, active support by) liberal and radical discourses in mainstream society. These discourses, traditionally available to colonized peoples as a main "route" out of oppression make this route more problematic for SLPs.

Second, the introduction of cochlear implant experimentation has led to scientific technology entering the Deaf domain on a major scale for the first time in Deaf history. One can argue that the advent of hearing aids actually constitutes the first example, but hearing aids were designed and sold mainly to deafened adults whereas the thrust of cochlear implant expansion has been directed at, and justified by, reference to Deaf children. Moreover, those who previously administered SLPs had some degree of contact with them. The current approach to childhood cochlear implantation relies on (and results in) a huge shift toward control being vested in scientific and biotechnology professionals who do not have, nor ever intend to have, contact with Deaf communities. Their exclusive interest is in biological and technological experimentation whose goals, objectives, and results are defined and assessed within a necessarily narrow range of definitions that do not require them to take into account any SLP discourses.

If the numbers of those professionals were small, that would be one thing. However, what is notable about the development of cochlear implantation is the extent of financial resources that have been invested in these experiments. The sums of money involved dwarf any other form of investment previously expended on the administration of SLPs. These resources have enabled the rapid spread of cochlear implantation, which has far outstripped the ability of groups opposed to the misuse of cochlear implants to demand full-scale, holistic, academic studies of the psychological, social, moral, and ethical consequences of such experiments, let alone achieve a moratorium. These financial issues are further examined later in this chapter. Given this background, how have the patterns of neocolonialism and cochlear implant experimentation played out in the United Kingdom?

Strategies and Patterns of Cochlear Implantation Development

Cochlear implantation in the United Kingdom has followed the same patterns as most Northern European countries, the United States, and Australia. Initial experiments were undertaken with adults during the early 1980s, followed by early experimentation with childhood implantation (in the mid-1980s), before any conclusive evidence of the benefits to adults was obtained.

Childhood implantation generally followed distinct stages:

- the implantation of deafened children;
- the implantation of children who were born deaf, subject to two basic criteria: a minimum age level and degree of hearing loss (criteria established in the late 1980s);
- the successive reduction of the minimum age for implantation to about the age of nine months (although implanting at later ages continues), which was reached about the late 1990s; and
- most recently, further reduction of the minimum age for implantation (to the age of five months) and bilateral implantation.

Christiansen and Barnartt (2003) report that cochlear implantation policies do vary among cochlear implant centers with respect to not only the above criteria but also the degree to which the use of sign language and involvement with Deaf communities is permitted during the process as well as the range of information (e.g., information about SLPs and their views) that is given to parents. Similar differences may occur in the United Kingdom but have not yet been the subject of research. Likewise, the number of Deaf children implanted in the United Kingdom is not available, but it appears that as many as 80 percent of all profoundly Deaf preschool children are now implanted.

It is important to understand how power structures operate within this form of neocolonialism. Although many teachers of Deaf children now accept the place of sign languages in education (see discussion that follows), the decision to implant a child is not within their control but is in the hands of the medical profession and preschool service providers who may seek to persuade parents to agree to implantation. Thus "liberal" teachers of Deaf children are faced with a fait accompli. In the face of these circumstances, they feel that their efforts are best expended by "adding" sign language to the lives of those children. The fact that these liberal teachers are introducing sign language to children in some situations should *not* be interpreted, as is so often the case, as a pluralistic approach (often described as "giving them the best of both worlds"). Adding signed language after implantation is the result of a rationalization based on the belief that this particular wave of neocolonialism cannot be halted. As will later become clear, permitting the Deaf child access to some sign language does not alter the fact that, in other crucial respects, their human rights have been breached. The design and promotion of the misuse of cochlear implantation as an intervention that "removes deafness" has led me and other opponents of implantation to label cochlear implantation an "Oralist approach" to SLPs, and this label applies whether or not signed language is permitted in the cochlear implantation process.

OPPOSING DISCOURSES: A BRIEF HISTORY

A brief summary of the history will frame the controversy for us. Deaf children were brought together to be educated in residential schools from the 1760s onward and, for the next century, were educated in their native (signed) languages. Deaf teachers, teaching assistants, and other auxiliary staff members worked alongside (if mostly under) hearing headmasters and hearing staff members. Research has not yet determined the point at which this process became colonialist, though a case can be made in Foucauldian terms for the structure always having been either colonialist or potentially colonialist (compare Ladd 2003, with respect to Irish Deaf education). However, the system became indubitably colonialist with the hegemony of Oralism after 1880.

The term *Oralism* is used here to describe an ideology whose fundamental goals are to remove anything "Deaf" from Deaf education, whether that be to ban sign language, remove Deaf teachers and other Deaf personnel, or erase any trace of Deaf cultural influence from Deaf children's lives (whether that influence occurs through curricula such as Deaf history and Deaf arts or through contact with the national Deaf community). It is important for the analysis undertaken in this chapter that the reader understand that Oralism is essentially a right wing, "conservative" discourse and a strategy driven by upper-class parents[2] of Deaf children (see, e.g., Lane 1984, 1993). One example of particular relevance to this chapter is Neisser's (1983) analysis of the Oralist Alexander Graham Bell Association:

> The chairman of the board of American Telephone and Telegraph (AT and T) [whose company actually deals in a wide range of electronic devices] traditionally sits on the board of the Bell Association. J. Edgar Hoover [head] of the FBI was a member for years. (31)

Despite more than two decades of organized protests by Deaf organizations and their allies between 1880 and 1900, Oralism gained hegemony and, during the twentieth century, consolidated its grip on each succeeding generation through an intensification of various colonialist strategies. The most important of these came with the advent of hearing aids, which enabled Oralists to halve potential SLP membership almost at a stroke, by creating the category of "partially hearing" and placing those children in mainstream schools.

It is also very important for any reader new to Deaf history to be aware that during this 100-year period, there was almost no nationwide research into the results of these policies until the work of Conrad (1979). The significance of this Oralist pattern of hegemony will be apparent as the chapter proceeds. When Oralism was finally challenged by researchers, proponents of Oralism refuted their research on the basis that the data analyzed were outdated and the results irrelevant because technological advances were now in widespread use—that there were now newer and better hearing aids, headphones, transmitters, and (eventually) cochlear implants. This standard line of argument to outsiders, whether to new parents or to the media, is of course very simple to maintain because technology is always advancing.

To understand the specific situation in the United Kingdom, one must recognize the overtly colonialist organizations that are the main players in this domain. As alluded to earlier, the British Deaf Association (BDA) became an arm of social welfare colonialism in the early twentieth century, and the National Deaf Children's Society (NDCS), a leading charity for Deaf children and their families in the United Kingdom, was set up as an arm of Oralist educational colonialism (Ladd 2003). However, a coordinating body was required to bring all deafness-related organizations together and in contact with the medical profession and relevant government bodies. Thus, the Royal National Institute of the Deaf (RNID) was established. About 1975, the RNID briefly passed through a liberal phase when it assisted with the process of evaluating the damage caused by Oralism by establishing seminars that were led by Conrad's (1979) preliminary research findings. But by the mid-1980s, it turned its attention back to facilitating the rapid spread of cochlear implantation programs and, since then, has been a major player in the process of their legitimization. The first Deaf chief executive officer of the RNID, Doug Alker, who was forced from office by Oralists in 1997, has written an in-depth account of how these processes are ruthlessly carried out (see Alker 2000). It should also be noted that more recently, the United Kingdom Council of Deafness (UKCOD) has been formed, establishing a further layer of neo-colonialist control and, in the process, defusing the growing Deaf movement toward decolonialism.

The Liberal Turn

The beginnings of the decolonization agenda are rooted in the 1970s. This agenda was partly a result of the broader social changes of the 1960s and partly influenced by Conrad and other researchers' revelations. Their studies exposed the damage enacted on Deaf children's education (literacy skills, in particular), mental health, and social functioning. Thus, these results became increasingly hard to disguise, and forms of sign language began to be accepted as a medium of instruction in many schools, although Deaf teachers were still not permitted in the education system. This "liberal" policy shift resulted in many Oralists leaving the schools and taking up posts within local authorities, ironically, having the effect of promoting them into positions of greater power because they now controlled the entrance of Deaf children into schools and preschools. By mainstreaming as many Deaf children as possible, they in effect starved the Deaf schools of their student population, forcing many into closure. Between 1934 and the present, the number of U.K. Deaf schools fell from 71 to fewer than 20 (Lee 2004). Of those still remaining, the numbers attending are miniscule compared with the past, and almost all of these schools may well close if action is not taken in the immediate future.

As stated earlier, the shift of the student population from Deaf schools to mainstream settings could not have been achieved without the "liberal" and "radical" discourses of the late 1980s that sought to mainstream children with a disability and insisted on classifying Deaf children within this category. As described earlier, because support for resistance to oppression is usually sought from those who ascribe to liberal or radical discourses, all avenues of resistance were now blocked to Deaf communities. The significance of this wave of neocolonialism was deeply felt because Deaf schools are the lifeblood of future SLPs and are the sites at which sign languages and Deaf cultures were learned (albeit surreptitiously during the period of Oralism). The danger for the quality of life of future community members was clear to those concerned with such qualities. Similar policies were enacted on Native Americans and Australian Aborigines during the twentieth century, cultural decimation through education being more significant than the usually suggested routes of enclosure onto reservations or poverty per se (Beresford and Omaji 1998; Churchill 2004).

Deaf Radicalism in the 1980s

In 1982, the radical U.K. Deaf organization, the National Union of the Deaf (NUD), developed a Charter of Rights for Deaf Children. The NUD examined the UN Charter and Universal Declaration of Human Rights created by the United Nations (UN) and sought recognition under such legislation, claiming that sign language communities constituted a linguistic minority (NUD 1982). It is useful to retrace the conceptual steps the NUD took:

- It examined the UN Rights of the Child and demonstrated that Oralism (and by implication cochlear implantation) breached all ten principles of the charter (NUD 1982, 34–48).
- It examined the Charter of Rights of the Disabled to illustrate how it offered no protection to Deaf children from Oralism because Deaf communities were, in fact, language minority communities (NUD 1982, 50–54).
- It located Article 27 of the UN International Covenant on Civil and Political Rights and outlined the ways in which Oralism breached this covenant, which states:

    In those States in which ethnic, religious or linguistic minorities exist, persons belonging to such minorities shall not be denied the right, in community with other members of their group, to enjoy their own culture, to profess and practice their own religion, or to use their own language.

- It located Articles that formally identify and categorize such breaches, notably the UN's Convention on the Prevention and Punishment of the Crime of Genocide. Article 2 of the convention lists the following five actions that constitute genocide:

  i. *killing members of the group;*
  ii. *causing serious bodily or mental harm to members of the group;*
  iii. *deliberately inflicting on the group conditions of life calculated to bring about its physical destruction, in whole or in part;*
  iv. *imposing measures designed to prevent births within the group; and*
  v. *forcibly transferring children of one group to another.*

  The NUD concluded that Articles 2–5 were breached by Oralism (NUD 1982, 56–61).
- It examined Article 3 of the UN's Convention on the Prevention and Punishment of the Crime of Genocide, which defines International Crimes by the following five acts: genocide itself, conspiracy to commit genocide, direct and public incitement to commit genocide, attempts to commit genocide, and complicity in genocide (NUD 1982, 61–64). The NUD concluded that Oralism was in breach of all five and that its practitioners should therefore be prosecuted under international law.

This campaign by the NUD to challenge the practices of Oralism by using international human rights conventions was unsuccessful largely because the UN could not conceive sign language communities as linguistic minorities, still perceiving them within the negative biology of disabled persons. Attempts to gain the support of the World Federation of the Deaf Congress in 1983 were suppressed by the WFD president (evidence of the internalized colonialism of Deaf leaders of the time).

With what we now know of the practices of cochlear implantation, it is possible to apply the NUD's analysis to the professions and persons involved in this process. Moreover, to the extent that government bodies, liberals, and radicals acquiesce in the process of cochlear implant experimentation, they too may be liable under the category of "complicity" cited above (see Article 3 of the UN's Convention on the Prevention and Punishment of the Crime of Genocide).

Given the heightened tone of Deaf radicalism in the early 1980s, it is no surprise that some Deaf organizations became actively concerned when the shift to implanting Deaf children began. The catalyst for action came when the Twentieth International Congress for Educators of the Deaf (ICED) took place in Manchester, United Kingdom, in 1985. It is important to note that the ICED was widely regarded as the most concentrated arm of colonialism, used since 1878 to legitimize Oralist policy with professionals and government and, thus, still one of the most visible means of promoting that legitimization through the media. The Second Congress, held in Milan in 1880, had become a symbol of colonialism for Deaf communities equivalent to the trope of "1492" for Native Americans and to the slave trade for African Americans. Moreover, Manchester was known to be the "home" of Oralism in the United Kingdom, that is, the center of its professional training programs.

The theme for the 1985 congress, proposed by the ICED organizing committee, was the issue they considered the most salient to Deaf education of the day—cochlear implants—which, at that time, had barely started to focus on implantation of children who were born Deaf. This decision ignited considerable opposition from both Deaf and hearing participants who considered several other issues to be far more important: the crisis of poor literacy levels, the pressing need to evaluate the role of signed language in Deaf education, and the need to consider when and how Deaf teachers should be permitted to return to the system.

The NUD and the North-West Region of the BDA came together in 1985 to mount the most extensive protests at an ICED Congress since the Paris Congress of 1900, where, after twenty years of organized Deaf protests, more than 200 Deaf teachers arrived, outnumbering the Oralists and, thus, were refused entry to the Congress.

Following the approach taken in Paris in 1900, an "Alternative Congress" was held at the Manchester Deaf Centre; protesters took to the streets for the first time that century, succeeding in getting the attention of the media, including a report on the protests on the British Broadcasting Corporation's main news program (*The Six O' Clock News*). As if to symbolize the resurgence of Deaf cultural issues, the famous and still active "Deaf Comedians Group" was formed to satirize the issues surrounding the ICED.

At that time, opposition raised by Deaf organizations against childhood implantation included the following key points:

- the experimental nature of childhood cochlear implantation when results on adults had not yet been fully reported,
- the child's inability to remove the cochlear implant,
- the immorality and breach of ethics that denied children the right to "decide for themselves when they are old enough whether they want to be experimented on," and
- the risk of long-term physical damage.

The Subsequent Decline of Deaf Opposition

The 1985 protests at the ICED Congress had thus developed the potential to halt the cochlear implant industry at an early stage; numerous newly opened doors now existed, not least of which was the media (the controversy assisting newspaper sales, of course). However, the momentum was lost in the years that followed. Run by a small group of volunteers, the NUD could not sustain a permanent campaign and passed the task on to the national organization that represented Deaf people in the United Kingdom, the BDA.

The BDA, only just emerging from its own (social welfare) colonialist roots, quickly passed the responsibility on to the NDCS. Formerly an Oralist organization, the NDCS was, at the time, run by pro-Deaf leadership. However, following the departure of that director, the Oralist succession in NDCS was restored. After the added blow of the demise of the NUD in 1987, Deaf opposition to cochlear implantation went underground once more.

It was not until 1994 that the BDA finally commissioned and produced a policy statement on cochlear implants, in response to continued pressure from grassroots membership. This document enlarged on the principles outlined previously in this section and raised concern that the parents of Deaf children might also be the victims of the cochlear implant industry. It also warned of the (hitherto unresearched) physical and other damage that might be caused to implanted children.[3] The campaign did not pursue the NUD's focus on the rights of the Deaf child under UN conventions, fearing that the term *genocide* was too emotive to be rationally understood by the average professional or government civil servant.

The campaign also did not focus on another important issue emerging at the time—the implantation of Deaf children who had previously been able to use hearing aids and whose hearing was subsequently destroyed by cochlear implant and replaced with the clearly inferior quality of sound produced by the implant. This issue is crucial when considering cochlear implantation in terms of human rights because if a child can hear by conventional means—that is, through hearing aids—then the grounds for implantation are removed, and the process is exposed for what it truly is: experimentation on Deaf children. Nevertheless, however worthy the BDA policy on cochlear implantation was, the momentum for the campaign had long been lost, and the BDA did little more than post copies of its policy and occasionally appear on radio programs when the issue of cochlear implantation was raised.

Cochlear Implants and Professional Silence

Mounting opposition to implantation was (and continues to be) severely handicapped by the success that the cochlear implant industry has had in maintaining professional silence around its work, in effect operating "below the radar." This process can be understood only if we also have an understanding of how neocolonialism operates; as emphasized earlier, in contrast to older approaches to colonialism, neocolonialism in the wider world (and in the Deaf world) operates out of sight of colonized populations. Because Deaf organizations were denied access to the subjects of childhood cochlear implantation, the only examples of the dangers and failures of cochlear implantation came to Deaf organizations from Deaf families who reported that they were subjected to unethical medical practices by being pressured to implant their own children.[4]

Teachers of Deaf children (even liberal teachers) declined to go on record about what they were seeing (a further example of the colonialist process at work). Parents, too, refused to speak out publicly. This silence is another vital human rights issue, and it is important that we understand why this silence might occur. First, as part of the colonialist process, parents have long been kept away from Deaf adults. Second, given that parents were aware of Deaf opposition to cochlear implantation, any operation that had gone wrong or failed to fulfill the promised outcomes filled parents with guilt and even shame. One can, therefore, understand that they sought to maintain a public silence. This point becomes especially relevant later in this chapter when I discuss the deaths of Deaf children that have occurred as a result of implantation and which were belatedly (and then only partially) revealed in 2002.

The Return of Organized Protests

The next protests against childhood cochlear implantation occurred in the United Kingdom in 1999. A small group of parents who did not want their children implanted joined with Deaf people in a series of lobbying efforts and protests. Although small and short-lived, these events were significant because they succeeded in getting considerable media attention. The media had become largely inured to the campaigning by SLPs themselves. But it seems that they thought the argument that some parents were happy with their Deaf children just the way they were born was a subject of potential controversy that would attract readers. This parent-inclusive approach has rarely been used since, but is clearly a strategy which offers a great deal of hope with regard to righting the imbalance of information disseminated to new parents.

Just before those 1999 protests, a new radical Deaf organization, the Federation of Deaf People (FDP) had been formed in 1998. Although opposed to implantation, its approach was to begin by campaigning for official government recognition of British Sign Language (BSL). That effort was seen as the first step in creating an Act of Parliament similar to the Welsh Language Act of 1993 that could ensure the protection of the sign language community as a collective entity. The intention in creating this Act was to focus on not only the individual rights of the Deaf child but also their collective rights as members of the sign language community. After a four-year battle during which the first-ever national "Deaf-plus-allies" marches took place, the government officially recognized BSL in March 2003.

The massive task of lobbying for legislation to follow up the recognition of BSL has yet to begin. One reason for the delay is the expectation that such legislation will bring a huge lobbying backlash from Oralists and cochlear implantation professionals, who of course have easy access to government as part of the colonizing arrangement. Taking on a hegemonic force of this size will require tremendous organizational and financial commitment from the traditionally impecunious BDA, FDP, and others. For these and other reasons, explicit campaigning against childhood cochlear implantation continues to be absent from the agenda set by those Deaf organizations.

Once again, as a result of Deaf grassroots dissatisfaction with the strategies adopted by existing Deaf organizations, another radical group was formed in 2001: the nonviolent, direct-action Deaf Liberation Front (DLF). The DLF organized protests at various meetings of cochlear implantation professionals, including an organized series of protests at the Seventh International Cochlear Implant Conference in Manchester in 2002. Despite being few in number, the information they researched and the reports they produced were significantly higher in quality than earlier literature protesting cochlear implants. The higher quality information helped achieve stronger media effects, but the major factor in their strong effort was a serendipitous release of information from the United States.

For the first time, information was released to the media about the deaths from meningitis of a number of child recipients of cochlear implants—indirectly the result of implantation. As each day passed, the number of reported deaths increased. Data from the U.S. Food and Drug Administration (FDA) Office of Surveillance and Biometrics were the first to emerge, reporting nine known deaths resulting from these cases. Surveys of cochlear implant centers were undertaken to identify additional, unreported cases. The FDA urged health professionals to report cases of implant recipients who had developed bacterial meningitis to MedWatch, the FDA's voluntary reporting program. As of May 2003, the FDA had identified 118 cases worldwide: 55 cases in the United States and 63 cases in other countries, patients ranging in age from 13 months to 81 years. Most U.S. patients were no older than five years (see U.S. FDA 2003). The United Kingdom reported no deaths, and implant manufacturers in other nations such as Australia were quick to distance themselves from the surgical procedures and particular implant device used in the United States.

It is important to note is that submission of this type of data was entirely voluntary. There was, and still is, no regulatory pressure to report all related deaths or, indeed, any related physical injuries in any country. Because only a small percentage of organizations responded voluntarily to the FDA, it is reasonable to assume that the damage (and consequent silence) is more extensive than so far admitted.[5] Furthermore, it appears that no centralized records of other medical complications or negative outcomes of implantation have been maintained. Although there have been several subsequent attempts to investigate the number of deaths related to cochlear implantation, almost all those investigations have been carried out by the cochlear implant industry itself.[6]

The DLF research also exposed the nature and extent of much of the world's current cochlear implant programming. A new feature of its campaign was to raise questions about whether there was any increased risk of cancer for cochlear implant recipients:

> There are . . . questions as to whether the device causes cancer in the same way as is alleged for mobile phones and overhead power lines. This is very scary when one considers that mobile phone users are not subjected to those electric currents 24 hours a day. (DLF 2002, 2)

Since 2002, DLF activities have been sporadic, with the latest protest occurring in May 2005 at a joint conference organized by The Ear Foundation (a U.K.-based cochlear implant charity), the RNID, and the NDCS. It appears that the conference organizing committee not only excluded Deaf community members from its organization but also discouraged Deaf people from giving keynote speeches or, indeed, presenting any papers at the conference (DLF 2005). Little or no attention was given in the conference to the issues of central importance to Deaf communities—the role of sign languages, Deaf culture, and Deaf teachers in education and so on. Instead, the focus was almost exclusively on the three neocolonialist waves described earlier—mainstreaming, cochlear implantation, and genetic modification (another reason why issues of cochlear implantation cannot be discussed in isolation from the other two neocolonialist waves).

In a clever move of the kind often used by other colonizing bodies, the conference was titled the "Deaf and Hearing Impaired Children Conference: Europe 2005." However, educators of Deaf children were not freely invited, and their official organizations were not invited to become part of any European alliance to support these children. The conference can be seen as an attempt by the cochlear implantation programmers to lay claim over Deaf education on a European-wide basis, gives an indication not only of the power and confidence the movement has attained but also of its future intent. Another indication of the colonizing intent of the organizers is the fact that this faux conference was held barely eight weeks before the next ICED Congress (a triennial event!).

Perhaps the organizers feared that ICED would be "too strongly" Deaf-focused and, therefore, took the preemptive step to establish an alternative power nexus. Ironically (or perhaps as another indication of the Oralist extremism of the cochlear implantation movement), the ICED turned out to be very "middle of the road," hosting a range of papers that expressed a range of views from Oralist to Deaf-focused. Even more ironic is the fact that the major sponsors of the ICED (without which the congress would not have been able to take place) were cochlear implant companies.[7] Thus, the penetration of powerful cochlear implant interests into Deaf education now goes much deeper than has previously been noted.

The Media and Conflicting Discourses

Two main media discourses can be identified: the discourse of mainstream television and newspapers and the discourse of the Deaf media. It is instructive to examine how these discourses have played out during the successive stages of the cochlear implantation movement.

Mainstream media focus on cochlear implantation by using several tropes. The first of these is the figurative term *miracle cure*, widely used to describe the anticipated outcomes of cochlear implants. That term is underpinned by a second, less explicit (more taken-for-granted) term, *progress*. When the media use this second term, the implied association is with science (for more on this connection, see Ladd 2003)—that social progress equates to scientific progress. Other media strategies include use of the term *bionic ear* (which becomes especially significant, as will be seen later) and the suggestion that Deaf communities are opposed to adult implantation. Thus, the public is faced with the sweeping exaggerations (in fact, outright lies) that somehow "deafness is now abolished"—a phrase used at the Milan Congress in 1880 and quoted in a major article in *The (London) Times* that very same week. In media appearances, Deaf people and their allies found that their time was thus mostly taken up by having to refute these red herrings rather than being able to focus on the experimentation and ethical arguments.

One argument that did receive airtime—though it was greeted with incredulity—was the view that "Deaf people are happy to be Deaf." The difficulty many hearing commentators had accepting this worldview was thus used to discredit the rest of the Deaf discourse—that cochlear implantation was experimental, that much damage was being caused and covered up, that Deaf children were experiencing human rights abuse, and so on (for a typical example, see Ladd 2003, 162).

It is particularly important to notice how neocolonialists position themselves in relation to these "over-claims" in the media. In private and in their daily work, they may suggest to parents and others that those claims are the result of exaggeration by public broadcasters. However, they may very well recognize the benefits they receive from these waves of media pressure on parents to "restore their child's hearing" and, therefore, can "have it both ways." This situation is all the more galling when the media continue their disinformation with, apparently, no intervention or correction by those who profit from the spin.

Televisual Discourses

The representation of cochlear implantation on television has followed the same pattern. An extra feature to note is the structure of television documentaries about cochlear implantation. Almost all programs focus on the events leading up to implantation, then end abruptly after the operation but before the results have been assessed. I know of no program that has followed up and has investigated the longer-term outcomes for cochlear implant recipients. Once again, such silence speaks volumes to the critical social scientist.

One particularly significant aspect of the 1999 parent-related protests mentioned above is that the media immediately became very interested in covering the issue. They had become inured to two decades of Deaf protests because of the pro-cochlear-implant spin that these were the actions of old-fashioned Deaf people fearfully "clinging to their own sickness." The advent of hearing parents who were happy for their child to be Deaf, some of whom actively wished for another Deaf child as companion to the first, was a revelation to the media, and press coverage from this angle was far easier to obtain. It is thus more the pity that very few Deaf organizations have formed coalitions with hearing parents of Deaf children from which a more powerful, media-attractive position could be established.[8]

Deaf Media Discourses

Although the Deaf print media have remained unequivocally opposed to childhood cochlear implantation, the response by Deaf television has been rather different. The main Deaf television program in the United Kingdom is the BBC's *See Hear,* which began in the 1980s with fairly evenhanded studio debates on the subject of cochlear implantation. A similar approach was taken by the United Kingdom's Channel 4 program, *Sign On.* By the mid-1990s, however, the position taken by *See Hear* and the United Kindgdom's newly established youth TV program, *Vee TV,* virtually endorsed cochlear implantation (Ladd 2007). Someone who is new to the Deaf community might suppose that Deaf television is Deaf controlled. This assumption would not be the case. Furthermore, Deaf television programs generally suffer from a major weakness: an almost total absence of investigative journalism. Because accurate representation of the cochlear implantation issue requires that solid investigative journalism be undertaken, those in Deaf television face even greater responsibilities to carry out quality journalism. In my view, however, the chance that Deaf television will strengthen its journalistic techniques is quite small.

THE FINANCIAL SCALE AND OTHER ASPECTS OF COCHLEAR IMPLANTATION PROGRAMS

It is now a common occurrence for conferences on deafness to be sponsored by cochlear implant organizations (and for delegates to receive all manner of cochlear implant advertising material in their conference satchels and to display related information prominently on conference name tags). The DLF's analysis of the financial backing of the 2002 Manchester conference was unable to identify a single delegate who had to pay for travel, conference registrations, or other expenses associated with the Congress (DLF 2002). That support was the result of just two cochlear implant organizations sponsoring the conference. By contrast, attendance by the roughly 10,000 attendees and speakers in 2002 at the *Deaf Way 2* conference in Washington, D.C., which involved a number of small sponsors, was, for the most part, at the attendees' own expense.

The cochlear implant industry is a multimillion dollar industry worldwide. One example of its vast wealth and reach can be seen in the events that took place during the first-ever Balkans conference on sign language in 2001. The conference took place at the time of a burgeoning sign language movement in Croatia. Much media attention was given to the newly "recognized" Croatian Sign Language, including coverage by the major national television news outlet. However, only a few months later, a huge push to implant Croatian Deaf children was launched, and the national newspapers and television networks were co-opted into action:

> It was the biggest humanitarian action in Croatia ever—"Let Them Hear." Around 2 million Euro were collected. TV presenters wear a big red badge with a logo and text "Let them hear." In the newspapers there is a whole page with a child's face and ear saying "she never heard Madonna—help her hear Madonna," or "He's never heard laughter—help him to hear laughter," to push people to call the telephone numbers. The final event was held in many cities and towns—famous singers and bands, sportsmen and politicians, even the president participated. . . . [E]ven mentally retarded, hard of hearing and autistic children are implanted. . . . [A]t the same time many children are dying because of heart disease (expensive operation), don't have money for wheelchairs, or dogs for the blind. (personal communication, hearing journalist, name withheld,[9] December 8 and December 22, 2001)

Clearly, immense power, influence, and resources were made available for this campaign (it may be instructive to note that Croatia has strong historical ties to Germany, a major cochlear implant player). Doubtless, this pattern will continue to be reproduced around the world. However, it does not end there.

The huge, ostensibly "global" financial investment in cochlear implantation is of special interest because very little profit is made by cochlear implant companies on the sale of an individual implant, and the number of Deaf children, in market terms, is minute. Given the greater potential for profit to be gained by targeting the larger section of the community who are hard of hearing or late-deafened adults, one must ask why the focus of attention is not more sharply directed to that group. Furthermore, given the small return to be gained from the immense amounts of money invested in the industry, how might these companies justify the small profit? One answer is that the money comes from the research and development (R & D) funds available to the industry. The next logical question to ask is, Is this money really being spent solely for the benefit of Deaf children?

Three sets of events at the 2002 Manchester conference brought these questions into focus. The first was the conference financing figures above, and the second was the huge imbalance in the type of papers presented. The third was that U.S. military personnel (in full uniform) were photographed attending the conference. Several possible explanations might clarify the reasons for their appearance, the first being that they were interested in the usefulness of cochlear implants for soldiers deafened in war (although as previously mentioned, late-deafened adults are not the industry's main focus). Another explanation, already considered by writers such as *Slate's*[10] deputy editor, David Plotz, is that the military may be using the interest in research on deafness as a stepping stone to super-normal hearing. For example, Plotz (2003) writes:

> The military is fascinated by the prospect that soldiers could learn to process more information more quickly. Can GIs, in essence, learn to hear faster? Information about this is hard to come by—none of the military scientists I phoned returned my calls—but according to civilian researchers I interviewed, the Air Force is studying it. . . . Research is current. The military may well be using the technology already. (n.p.)

However it is also possible the military might have become interested in the use of Deaf children as an experimental way station en route to other, more far-reaching goals.

To understand the military's presence more fully, one should be aware that it has long been a matter of record that the U.S. military has been experimenting with electromagnetic technology for warfare purposes (see Welsh n.d.) and that this experimentation has been one of the driving forces behind the development of the fields of nanotechnology and biotechnology. Many companies and universities involved in this work have conducted and financed both civilian and military R & D.

One of the most active areas of work is called the "brain-machine interface," which considers the usefulness to both civil and military society of a wide range of human implants, including the cochlear implant. This field is more widely known as bionics. A comprehensive summary of the range of bionics can be found in a document assembled by the European Group on Ethics in Science and New Technologies for the European Commission, titled "Ethical Aspects of ICT Implants in the Human Body" (Rodotà and Capurro 2005).

Sidney Perkowitz, professor of physics at Emory University in Atlanta, discusses cochlear implants in his article "Becoming Bionic" (about the benefits and dangers of bionics) and states:

> Although much current research in bionics is motivated by medical applications, a good deal of the work in the U.S. is sponsored by the Department of Defense, which wants to make soldiers more effective through such means as direct neural control of weaponry. (Perkowitz 2005)

Direct neural control is also related to brainstem research, which is another burgeoning development, an offshoot of cochlear implant research.

In an article published in *OHSU* (the Oregon Health and Science University magazine), Professor Jan van Santen, professor and head of the Center for Spoken

Language Understanding at the School of Science and Engineering, confirms Perkowitz's (2005) assessment of the military link:

"[S]peech technology has traditionally been driven by the military and tele-communications industries," said van Santen, a longtime Bell Labs researcher who joined the School of Science & Engineering in 2001. (Oregon Health and Science University 2002, n.p.)

The earliest reference yet found that shows a connection between cochlear implants and the military comes from *Spinoff*, an annual publication of the National Aeronautics and Space Administration (NASA)[11] that features successful partnership benefits. The journal records:

In 1977, NASA helped Kissiah obtain a patent for the cochlear implant. Several years later he sold the rights of the technology to a company named BIOSTIM. (NASA 2003, n.p.)

A more recent example can be found in *The Journal* (news and information for national naval medical center personnel, published by DCMilitary.com) where an article praising cooperation among traditional rival services to implant Deaf children asserts:

[The] Army and Navy work together in unison to achieve a common goal. . . . [Doctor CDR McKinnon] also stressed the importance and cost-effectiveness for performing the procedure on hearing-impaired children. . . . "A child will save $50,000 over his [sic] lifetime by having the procedure," McKinnon said. (Walz 2005, n.p.)

A similar example of the ease with which these fields now converge can be found in the University of Michigan's development of the "mechanical cochlea."[12] A university press release states: "The 3-centimeter device could potentially be used as part of a cochlear implant. More immediate applications include a low-power sensor for military or commercial applications" (University of Michigan 2005).

Just as Plotz (2003) found, confirming the explanation that the military could be using cochlear implant research to further their own goals in bionics may be impossible. At the very least, it would require committed investigative journalism. In recent decades, we have witnessed the emergence of the "military industrial complex" (a term coined by U.S. President Eisenhower in 1961) in which electronics and other new technologies are developed by companies working for both the private and military sectors; to this extent, government funding can be used to subsidize the loss-making private sector. If the money trail could be followed, it may just lead to companies of this kind and it may be possible to identify from which sector the R & D funds originated. In raising this issue, it is not my intention to suggest that the United States alone might be involved in such practices. Companies of this kind are often multinational entities, and the web of involvement may cross national boundaries. Given the absence of the kind of investigative journalism that is needed to confirm or reject such suggestions, it appears that SLPs are not yet important enough to the liberal and radical discourses. If they were, then just the smallest amount of evidence would be enough to spark a tabloid frenzy: "Deaf Children Experimented on for Military Purposes" might be the least sensational of the headlines.

A precedent exists for the potential turnaround that is possible in public opinion: the issue of genetically modified foods in 1999. In less than three weeks, U.K. media headlines shifted from condemnation of the Luddites who were destroying the possibility of bionic, germ-free food to outright condemnation of "Frankenstein food." Consequently, public opinion also did a 180-degree turn within a matter of weeks.

The Place of Deaf Studies in Cochlear Implantation Discourses

Until the 1970s, those who refuted Oralism had little or no support from academic researchers. Not until the 1970s did educational research into deafness start in earnest, followed by the emergence of sign linguistics. Linguistic recognition that sign languages were bona fide languages enabled not only the crucial conceptual foundation for the Deaf movements (described above) to be set in place but also the formal establishment of Deaf Studies as a discipline.

Over the last fifteen years, Deaf Studies curricula and research centers around the world have had the potential to expose (by impartial research) the actions occurring within, and the consequences of, mainstreaming plus cochlear implantation. This potential, by and large, has not materialized. First, around the world, very few Deaf Studies courses even teach on the subject of cochlear implantation; at best, it may form part of a single teaching unit. Therefore, students of Deaf Studies have had limited opportunity to develop a discourse about these topics or to generate clear theoretical perspectives that can be taken out into the wider world and used to argue the Deaf view.

The second obstacle to using the potential of Deaf Studies courses to address cochlear implantation issues is the difficulty that established researchers have experienced in gaining funds for research or projects in this field. For example, researchers who have been highly successful obtaining funding for other projects reportedly have difficulty attracting support for projects that investigate the psychological and social effects of cochlear implantation. The reason for this difficulty becomes clear when we realize that, in general, applications for research projects are sent for refereeing to a panel of specialists in the field to which the research pertains. Therefore, applications for research into cochlear implantation are usually sent to "cochlear implant specialists" who may be employees of the cochlear implant industry or who otherwise have positions that are subsidized or supported by the industry.

The assessment of the psychological and social effects of cochlear implantation is important information that needs to be made available to cochlear implant practitioners (see Preisler, this volume). However, the field's limited interest in this kind of research suggests that such information may be seen to threaten cochlear implantation programs; certainly, some of this research would challenge the hegemony of cochlear implant practitioners and question their claim as sole adjudicators of what constitutes valid research in this field.

Research funding is also difficult to obtain for the investigation of rejection rates by Deaf children who refuse to use the devise after implantation and for any negative consequences of implantation. Minimal research on rejection rates has been undertaken (Lane 1993) or made available in the public domain. Despite the importance of such statistics and the usefulness to implant teams to understand the reasons for a Deaf child's rejection of an implant, it appears that this area of research is discouraged.

Similarly, negative experiences of deafened adults who have been implanted appear on consumer Web sites and in online chat rooms but are rarely the subject of academic research. Perusal of these experiences reveals numerous cases of multiple physical symptoms and other negative consequences of implantation, but these are not shared with practitioners or acted on. For example, one such sufferer gave the following reason for the silence of those experiencing negative symptoms:

> [Otherwise,] the Deaf culturalists will try to claw the entire CI [cochlear implantation] programme out of consideration [sic], by distortion, innuendo, misleading statistics and outright lies. (online chat room participant, name withheld for the purpose of anonymity)

Such a position might seem reasonable were it not for the fact that the walls of silence described throughout this chapter actually make the "distortion, innuendo, misleading statistics, and outright lies" easy for the cochlear implant industry to get away with. Clearly, adult implantees also need to become the subject of independent research.

The situations described above are all reasons why those who are involved in developing and teaching Deaf Studies programs may need to make more effort to contribute to research on cochlear implantation. As matters stand, the overwhelming numbers of studies undertaken on any aspect of cochlear implantation are produced within the industry by those involved in cochlear implantation programs in hospitals, universities, or science laboratories. Very little truly independent research currently exists. The DLF research on the 2002 Manchester conference identified 530 presentations of which

- none were by Deaf organizations or parents' organizations,
- four questioned the experimental nature of the work,
- seventeen addressed physical side effects of the experiments, and
- one addressed psychological and social effects.

Thus, the other 508 conference presentations responded to the narrowest of self-defined industry parameters.

A further challenge for those in the Deaf Studies field is to confront the assertion that cochlear implantation is a "cure" for deafness. That assertion has become so all-pervasive that minimal thought has been given to the existential and phenomenological reality for a child whose implant is "successful"—that is, for a child who can function as a hard of hearing person when the device is worn and switched on. The assumption made in this idea of a successful implantation is that being hard of hearing is preferable to being Deaf. However, a considerable number of personal testimonies from Deaf people and deaf people who are not a part of the Deaf community, all of whom were raised orally or were mainstreamed into hearing schools, challenge this view (compare Taylor and Bishop 1991; Taylor and Darby 2003; DEX 2003). These testimonies contain moving accounts of coming from a state of "lostness" in the mainstream to finding the "light" and "coming home" when the signing Deaf community is discovered. The sheer volume of these accounts, just the tip of the iceberg in terms of the real numbers involved, effectively draws into question any assumption that for a person to be deaf (or Deaf) and to forced to live as one who is hard of hearing, mainstreamed, and assimilated is a desirable state of existence.

Again, one might expect the cochlear implant industry to consider this subject worthy of research, but because it does not, the responsibility falls to the field of Deaf Studies to give priority to seeking research funding to undertake in-depth studies of this kind. The information such studies may reveal is crucial for informing hearing parents, thus enabling them to reach more unbiased decisions than they are currently able to do when faced with the pressure of only medical and Oralist discourses.

Emerging "Liberal" Cochlear Implantation Discourses

The emerging "liberal" cochlear implantation discourses comprise three main aspects: the issue of implants plus sign language, a key shift in the nature of the discourses, and the "subculturation" of a new group of adult implantees. Analysis of these discourses reveals their interconnections among cochlear implantation, mainstreaming, and genetic modification and, thus, the importance of considering the other waves of neocolonialism when critiquing cochlear implantation.

The first of the liberalizing cochlear implantation discourses, implants plus signed language, is becoming the modus operandi in some countries. In Scandinavia and most of the United States, for example, Deaf schools still operate with significant numbers of children, so their existence is not yet overtly threatened and there is rarely any focus on the possibility of a threat. However, this reality is not the situation in the United Kingdom and elsewhere, as noted earlier. The remaining Deaf schools in the United Kingdom, most of which follow a bilingual educational model (some taking further steps toward decolonization), are in serious danger of closure. The reason is simple. Preschools' programs are able to make the (false) argument that having a cochlear implant equates with becoming hard of hearing and, thus, with being able to be successfully mainstreamed. This position takes no account of the difficulties and dangers for those who have had negative experiences of mainstreaming. Indeed, such concerns are seen as secondary to the need to swiftly implant and transfer those Deaf children into the mainstream and to then close the Deaf schools before serious questions can be asked, thus preventing any going back. Once closed, the schools cannot easily be reestablished.[13]

The second aspect of liberalism is the shift in Deaf discourses, particularly in the United States. For the first time, a growing number of adults in the Deaf community are themselves obtaining an implant. This new group of implant recipients appears to be largely made up of either those who were deafened in childhood and wish to take the chance of reexperiencing what they once knew or those who remained particularly oral—that is, who continued to be somewhat in thrall to their childhood model. In classic postcolonial literature, equivalent members of the latter group are said to be continuing to experience "colonization of the mind."[14]

As with any other colonized group, the Deaf community initially condemned those among them who so overtly demonstrated what was perceived as "disloyalty" to the group. However, this development has occurred at the same time as the first generation of implantees has reached college age. At the National Technical Institute for the Deaf (NTID) in Rochester, for example, as many as 10 percent of the 2,000 students (most of whom graduated from mainstream programs) wear cochlear implants. The number is expected to rise sharply over the next decade given the industry's continuing market penetration. The fact that these students attended a Deaf university is of course an indication that cochlear implantation programs have not been fully successful in persuading these students that they can (and should) assimilate into mainstream society.

Nevertheless, their attending NTID does not mean that they have escaped "unscathed." Because they were not fully enculturated into the Deaf community during childhood, they can expect a difficult rite of passage. Without a specially designed Deaf Studies program made available during their education, the danger remains that they may form a subgroup or subculture within the Deaf community without the opportunity to fully contribute to, and benefit from, local, national, and international Deaf communities. It is this process of "subculturation" as much as their disappearance from the Deaf community that threatens the transmission of knowledge about the Deaf world and is the third aspect of the "liberal" discourse. That 250-year-old body of cultural history, knowledge, values, and traditions of the SLPs are the sum total of the lessons and triumphs of Deaf people, the positive biology described at the outset of this chapter.

Further Effects of Neocolonialism on Deaf Communities

Previous sections in this chapter describe problems being created for the U.K. Deaf community. One of the most serious relates back to the combination of cochlear implantation and mainstreaming. Note also that many Deaf schools struggle to offer the education they wish to because, after the effects of mainstreaming, they are left with a higher percentage of less able and multiply disabled children. Ironically, one feature that helps keep some Deaf schools alive is the incursion of "mainstream failures"—students from age 11 upward, who come back to Deaf schools. Unfortunately, because many of these children are damaged by their prior experience, they tend to drag down the education that can be offered to the able, bilingually raised children.

These developments are compounded because the number of parents with implanted children is reaching a "critical mass." Parents who have chosen to adopt the Deaf community's position on cochlear implantation often report (anecdotally) that they face growing pressure from other parents who have been known to make remarks such as "If you really loved your child, you would give him (or her) an implant." In actuality, many of these parents have taken considerable pains, including giving up their jobs and moving to another part of the country, to choose a powerful and positive education for their child in a bilingual school for Deaf students, one that brings them and their children in contact with Deaf adults and, sometimes, with the Deaf community. Given that this kind of education is the same kind that should not have been stopped 120 years ago, the imminent closures of schools for the Deaf in the United Kingdom are nothing short of a disaster.

There are numerous examples of the negative effects of the waves of neocolonialism on Deaf people, but one of the most recent is the intervention of the judicial system into issues surrounding Deaf identity. There have been cases reported in the United Kingdom, United States, and Australia of the courts (a) determining whether or not a child will be implanted against the wishes of one or more parent (see Mills, this volume), (b) attempting to force Deaf couples to implant their own children (see Hall 2002), and (c) not allowing Deaf children to be fostered or adopted unless first implanted. These are staggering developments, especially when considering that judicial review might be more appropriately focused on determining the extent to which these decisions constitute child abuse (compare NUD 1982; earlier this chapter).

At this point, mention must be made of the third wave of neocolonialism, genetic modification. Genetic modification lurks in the background as a (semiconcealed) next scenario, another example of negative biology, and potentially as the "final solution" for Oralism. All that is happening in the cochlear implantation field is now taking place within the larger context of soon-to-appear developments in genetic modification, which manifests itself in two ways. One is that Oralists are again able to assert that SLPs and Deaf cultures will disappear into history and therefore "resistance is futile."

The second way involves the implication that, because of the sheer size and scale of the new biotechnological industrial complex, the cochlear implant industry may likely make an easy transition to becoming involved in genetic modification (a continuum of technological "advancement"). Indeed, evidence suggests that this transition is already taking place. The Australian inventor of the multichannel cochlear implant, Professor Graeme Clark, recently announced, with the Bionic Ear Institute and other collaborators, their move into research on other neural prostheses such as nerve regrowth for spinal cord injury (The Bionic Ear Institute 2005). It is now clear that what was seen as two separate waves of neocolonialism (cochlear implantation and genetic modification) is part of an all-encompassing tide. Thus, the kind of arguments and strategies needed to resist genetic modification need to be considered and applied to the present situation of cochlear implantation.

So, what might these arguments be? Clearly, SLPs have to "move up a gear" and formulate a positive defense to the question of the legitimacy of their very existence—that is, why Deaf peoples should be allowed to continue to exist in human form. To create this defense, the Deaf world must stress its contribution to human knowledge and the world at large. In short, leaders in the Deaf world must explore and publicly debate all aspects of the positive biology concept (another role and arguably a priority for Deaf Studies courses).

This chapter has demonstrated that the cochlear implantation wave of neo-colonization may be in breach of statutory legislation and international conventions. The question thus remains, why are these supposed breaches not being directly challenged by Deaf organizations and their allies?

THE DEAF RESURGENCE

One reason why Deaf organizations and their allies are not directly challenging what is happening is historically rooted. At this time, the national and international "Deaf Resurgence" (see Ladd 2003 for a definition and description), having just emerged from a century-long suppression, is focused on internally rebuilding its cultures and on reconstructing positive education systems. These efforts have resulted in a huge expansion of cultural, artistic, and professional activities now accessible to the increasing numbers of Deaf professionals. The net result is that energies are diffused, and talented young Deaf leaders who would otherwise be most profitably employed as activists within national Deaf organizations have numerous other doors open to them. This situation is compounded by the fact that such organizations themselves are only just beginning to move (if they are moving at all) out of the colonialist mentality of meek acceptance and mild protest.

Such cultural submission and conservatism runs deep. The process to change from a social organization to a radical political body meets with much resistance. Within Deaf cultures, there is still a deep fear of "offending" hearing people. SLPs have, broadly speaking, not had access to information available to hearing people through television, radio, cinema, theater, books (because of Oralism), and the workplace—information suggesting that the status quo can be challenged. Indeed, there has been little awareness that, throughout history, there have been groups and individuals who challenged and surmounted discrimination, marginalization, and other imposed disadvantages.

Ironically, the response from hearing people trained through Deaf Studies programs is one of respect for, yet a hands-off attitude toward, the SLPs' struggle for self-determination (which is a logical reaction because they are conscious of the history of paternalism and control over Deaf people by their hearing predecessors). Their knowledge of the majority culture, however, is very much needed. They have an important role to play as allies as Deaf communities face the huge task of redefining their place in society. But this postcolonial development has not yet been acknowledged, and until it is, this traditionally important route for oppressed groups—gaining allies from the majority society—remains virtually dormant.

Cochlear Implants and Legislation Options

Assuming that efforts could be made to call for a moratorium on cochlear implants until proper independent research could be carried out, on what basis and in which domains might these efforts be made? At least four options are available.

1. *The linguistic minority recognition option.* Existing campaigns to attain official recognition and protection of sign languages must continue. It may be that

such recognition needs to take precedence over other options to persuade international bodies such as the UN that sign language communities should be recognized as "linguistic minorities" rather than as disability groups.

2. *The genocide option.* After (or even together with) the official recognition of sign languages and sign language communities, the NUD's strategy of using the UN conventions could be adopted. Parallel actions could be taken with respect to regional bodies such as the European Court of Human Rights, the European Union, and so on.

3. *The child abuse option.* Those seeking to undertake more immediate anti-cochlear-implantation campaigns might, more fruitfully, focus on existing national and regional legislation to prevent child abuse. Working in tandem with Deaf Studies programs, efforts could be made to show how Oralist cochlear implantation programs and mainstreaming can be considered under such legislation.

4. *The financial reparations option.* A strategy that has worked well in other domains (because most major industries are capitalist in nature) is to sue for damages of one kind or another. If cases were won, such as occurred in the tobacco industry, then the cochlear implant and Oralism industry would, in all likelihood, pull back from policies that may expose them to further potential financial risk, negative publicity, or both. A classic case with direct relevance to the situation involves the efforts by more than 200,000 women worldwide who are battling for compensation for injury from silicone breast implants. On September 10, 2002, a ten-year legal battle ended for 3,100 Australian women in the Victorian Supreme Court; final payments were approved from a $35 million fund, successfully claimed from Dow Corning, a breast implant company (Pheasant 2002). Some cases have been (halfheartedly) brought against local education authorities, for example, by parents whose children grew up Oralist and now cannot read or write. But inappropriate organization within the Deaf community and lack of support from allies (including lack of media attention) has enabled judges to dismiss such cases. The outcomes of these cases could have been legally challenged, but often, limited financial resources or colonialist legal advice proves too great an obstacle. Nevertheless, this route is open to any determined group of people who wish to take such matters to, say, the European Court of Human Rights (whose decisions are actually legally binding on member state judiciaries).

Preempting the Genetic Modification Wave

Ultimately, it is the genetics wave that must be defeated. Deaf communities may survive cochlear implantation, however badly damaged; but genetic modification, by definition, intends for them not to survive at all.[15] Seeking legal protection under language minority rights legislation seems the most appropriate action to take against genetic modification because attempts to enact genetic modification programs can be identified as having the intention to remove the world's 250-plus native signed languages—a much clearer legal position to defend.

Unlike the first two waves of neocolonialism, mainstreaming and cochlear implantation, taking on the genetic modification movement offers the possibility for alliances and coalitions to be formed beyond the Deaf domain. There are six obvious sets of potential allies for such a campaign. For each group, a different line of approach needs to be taken, and different concepts and tropes invoked.

1. *The green movement.* Using positive biology is an ideal strategy with groups in the green movement, given their emphasis on respecting naturalism (see Ladd 1998). Forming alliances with these groups will take considerable relationship building because Deaf communities are currently distant from those in the green movement.

2. *Religious groups.* These groups constitute an important source of potential alliances, partly because of their numbers, partly because of their social status, and partly because they are (generally) culturally conservative; that is, their social circles are more likely to overlap with those of some Deaf people, for example, Deaf Christians. It is also possible to demonstrate Biblical evidence of God's support for the continued existence of Deaf peoples (see, e.g., Exodus 4:11, Leviticus 19:11, Psalm 19:1–4, and Psalm 94:8–10).

3. *Gay, lesbian and feminist hearing groups.* This source of support (stimulated by genetic modification attempts to "find the gay gene") is potentially very powerful. Relationships between Deaf communities, and gay and lesbian hearing communities are the best example of Deaf-hearing social relationships. Indeed, these communities offer a model to majority societies with respect to including, as opposed to assimilating, SLPs.

4. *Other minority groups.* These groups range from ethnic minorities (such as the Welsh) to religious minorities. Therefore, a range of strategies may be needed to make contact and gain support.

5. *Disability groups.* The Deaf Resurgence's ideology espousing "linguistic minority, not disability," together with anger toward pro-assimilation disabled activists who gained control of the disability movement (and are thus complicit in Deaf school closure), has led to a political gulf between the two groups. Consequently, the truly radical aspects of Disability Studies have mostly been excluded from Deaf community and Deaf Studies domains. Ironically, people with disabilities, like those in signing communities, are also under threat from genetic modification; unlike the latter, however, they have already vigorously organized themselves.[16] Deaf peoples can easily cultivate this source of alliance if they move beyond "knee-jerk" reactions and realize the potential of working alongside disability groups to attain decolonization.

6. *Parents of Deaf and disabled children.* In most countries, these parents remain a tremendously underused asset. It is of major importance that parents who

have positive feelings toward their Deaf children, whether young or grown, be asked at the very least to submit testimonials and, hopefully, to become more politically engaged with the community to which they, in part, belong.

Members of several of the groups mentioned above are already working with politicians in a coalition focused on bioethics, notably Disabled Peoples' International. The current political benchmark for what has been achieved so far is the set of documents adopted at the 1999 United Nations Educational, Scientific and Cultural Organization (UNESCO) Conference on Sciences (see UNESCO 2002).

A formidable coalition thus has the potential to come into being. Perhaps the beauty of undertaking such a task in these dark and unpromising times is the life-affirming, Deaf-celebrating nature of the praxis. The arguments for positive biology (together with the research and teaching required to support them) mean that the educative process of coalition building can be positive and pleasurable. The focus on this work will be one of appreciation because in the face of more than a century of oppression, we still continue to witness the remarkable survival and achievements of the Peoples of the Eye.

Notes

1. The domains and eras involved in this analysis are extensive, so the chapter at times must use generalizations where necessary to illustrate underlying patterns.
2. By contrast, multiculturalism and linguistic diversity are generally seen as attributes of left wing politics.
3. Among the numerous negative physical effects of cochlear implantation, one has barely been considered because it has only recently been discovered in the wider medical field. That effect is vestibular illness, which sometimes results from operations to the head, but whose severe effects may not kick in until a decade or more later.
4. Two examples will suffice. One family in which the father was Deaf and the mother was a child of Deaf adults (known as a CODA) reported that when the father left the room, attempts were made to persuade the mother to accept the cochlear implantation. Another Deaf couple, who refused cochlear implantation for their child, found that the doctors contacted the hearing grandparents and asked them to put pressure on the Deaf couple. The latter is of course a clear example of a breach of ethics related to patient confidentiality.
5. During the week of the DLF protests, the protesters were approached during one midnight vigil by a French doctor who informed them that he knew that the numbers of deaths stated on the DLF leaflets was actually considerably higher.
6. The DLF and others have talked of the need to identify those Deaf children who have died and to hold vigils at their graves. This potentially media-powerful intention has so far been stymied by the difficulty in obtaining this information.
7. A considerable number of delegates complained that the identity tags they had to wear for the week were covered with the "C" word!
8. We should also study the ways in which the media respond to genetically related Deaf issues if we are to understand how best to respond to the cochlear implantation debate. The best example to date is the 2002 *Washington Post Magazine* article (Mundy

2002) about a Deaf lesbian couple who chose to have a second Deaf child through artificial insemination and the way that the originally very balanced story was misrepresented when it went across the wire to other media outlets (see, e.g., Giese 2002; Langton 2002; Tsavdaridis and Hailstone 2002).

9. Names have been withheld in this section to protect the anonymity of the sources, as requested.

10. *Slate* is an award-winning online news association.

11. On NASA's Scientific and Technical Information homepage (http://www.sti.nasa.gov/STI-public-homepage.html, accessed January 19, 2006), readers are directed to *Spinoff* to "Find out how NASA research affects everyday life here on Earth."

12. If so, Wrigley's (1996) case for the emergence of a cybernetic mindset becomes salient.

13. This Oralist attitude even permeates at least one U.K. bilingual school, where it is reported that some parents with cochlear implants do not bother to learn to sign even within the bilingual environment. Another alarming development is the assertion that the families of numerous would-be implantees have to sign a contract agreeing to a nonsigning school program before operations can go ahead.

14. It is instructive to notice here how hard the media had to look to find the (very few) examples of Deaf families desiring implants. Although the 1999 U.S. television documentary *Sound and the Fury* (Aronson 2001, 2006) sought to present a pro-cochlear-implant perspective, it was obvious to my own graduate students that a very powerful hearing grandmother was instrumental in creating the pressure on the Deaf family. This aspect of the documentary echoes the situation of the medical focus on hearing grandparents in an earlier footnote—clearly, a recurring, though little-noticed phenomenon.

15. A chilling example (in its absurdity) of what is to come was recently reported in *The Independent London* (Lichfield 2005). The article, headed "Disabled have right not to be born, court rules," noted that the court protestors said this position was a legally sanctioned step toward eugenics, or selected breeding.

16. Visit the Web sites (all accessed January 19, 2006) of Disabled Peoples' International (http://www.dpi.org) and the United Kingdom's Disability Awareness in Action (http://www.daa.org.uk), and see the work of disabled academics like Gregor Wolbring, an advisor on bioethics to the Council of Canadians with Disabilities (http://www.euthanasiaprevention.on.ca/Articles/gregorwolbring/gwolbring.htm).

References

Alker, D. 2000. *Really not interested in the deaf?* Darwen, Lancashire, United Kingdom: Darwen Press.

Aronson, J. 2001. *Sound and fury.* New York: Aronson Film Associates and Public Policy Productions.

———. 2006. *Sound and fury: Six years later.* http://www.pbs.org/wnet/soundandfury.

Beresford, Q., and P. Omaji. 1998. *Our state of mind: Racial planning and the stolen generations.* South Fremantle, Australia: Fremantle Arts Centre Press.

The Bionic Ear Institute. 2005. *Strategic directions: 2005–2015.* Melbourne: The Bionic Ear Institute. http://www.bionicear.org/bei/BEI_Strategic_Directions.pdf.

Christiansen, J. B., and S. N. Barnartt. 2002. *Deaf president now! The 1988 revolution at Gallaudet University.* Washington, D.C.: Gallaudet University Press.

———. 2003. *Cochlear implants: Ethics and choices*. Washington, D.C.: Gallaudet University Press.

Churchill, W. 2004. *Kill the indian, save the man*. San Francisco: City Lights Books.

Conrad, R. 1979. *The deaf school child: Language and cognitive function*. London: Harper and Row.

Crouch, B. A. 1941/1998. The people of the eye. Repr. *Reviews in American History*, 26 (2): 402–07.

Deaf Ex-Mainstreamers Group (DEX), ed. 2003. *Between a rock and a hard place*. Wakefield, United Kingdom: DEX.

Deaf Liberation Front (DLF). 2002. Press pack, issued September 3. London: DLF.

———. 2005. Press release, issued May 24. Preston, United Kingdom: DLF.

Deloria, V. 1988. *Custer died for your sins*. Norman, Okla.: Oklahoma University Press.

Giese, R. 2002. Are we playing God with kids? Lesbian couple who sought out deaf sperm donor are fulfilling desires of all would-be parents. *The Toronto Star*, April 18, A31.

Hall, J. 2002. Mich. judge rules deaf boys needn't undergo surgery. *The Boston Globe*, May 10, A3.

Jankowski, K. A. 1997. *Deaf empowerment: Emergence, struggle, and rhetoric*. Washington, D.C.: Gallaudet University Press.

Ladd, P. 1998. The green movement and signing communities. Paper presented at "Green Future" workshop, Glastonbury Festival, June 26–28, Glastonbury, Somerset, United Kingdom.

———. 2003. *Understanding deaf culture*. Clevedon, United Kingdom: Multilingual Matters.

Ladd, P. 2007. Signs of change—Sign language and televisual media in the U.K. In *Minority language media: Concepts, critiques and case studies*, ed. M. Cormack and N. Hourigan. Cleveden, U.K.: Multilingual Matters.

Ladd, P., and D. West. Forthcoming. *Deafhood pedagogies—Deaf educators and the unrecognised curriculum*. New York: Oxford University Press.

Lane, H. 1984. *When the mind hears: A history of the deaf*. New York: Vintage Books.

———. 1993. *The mask of benevolence*. New York: Random House.

Langton. J. 2002. Lesbians: We made our baby deaf on purpose. *The Evening Standard*, April 8.

Lee, R., ed. 2004. *A beginner's introduction to deaf history*. Feltham, United Kingdom: British Deaf History Society Publications.

Lichfield, J. 2005. Disabled have right not to be born, court rules. *The Independent London*, April 20.

Malzkuhn, M., J. Covell, G. Hlibok, and B. Bourne-Firl. 1994. Deaf president now. In *The deaf way: Perspectives from the international conference on deaf culture*, ed. C. J. Erting, R. C. Johnson, D. L. Smith, and B. D. Snider, 829–37. Washington, D.C.: Gallaudet University Press.

Mottez, B. 1993. The deaf mute banquets and the birth of the deaf movement. In *Looking back*, ed. R. Fischer and H. Lane, 143–56. Hamburg: Signum.

Mundy, L. 2002. A world of their own. *Washington Post*, March 31, W22.

National Aeronautics and Space Administration (NASA). 2003. Hearing is believing. *Spinoff 2003*, n.p. http://www.sti.nasa.gov/tto/spinoff2003/hm_3.html.

National Union of the Deaf. 1982. *Charter of rights of the deaf, part one: The deaf child.* London: National Union of the Deaf.

Neisser, A. 1983. *The other side of silence.* Washington, D.C.: Gallaudet University Press.

Oregon Health and Science University. 2002. Deaf children learn to talk using speech technology from OGI School of Science & Engineering: Computer serves as friendly tutor for children at Portland's Tucker Maxon School. *OHSU News and Information,* June 3. http://www.ohsu.edu/unparchive/2002/060302hearing.html.

Perkowitz, S. 2005. Becoming bionic. *Emory Magazine,* n.p. http://www.emory.edu/EMORY_MAGAZINE/spring_2005/bionic.html.

Pheasant, B. 2002. Final implants payments approved. *The Financial Review,* September 11, 9.

Plotz, D. 2003. Hearing aid: Is there a better ear? *Slate,* March 10. http://www.slate.com/id/2079181.

Rodotà, S., and R. Capurro. 2005. Ethical aspects of ICT implants in the human body: Opinion 20, European Group on Ethics in Science and New Technologies. Paper presented to the European Commission, March 16. http://ec.europa.eu/european_group_ethics/docs/avis20compl.pdf.

Taylor, G., and J. Bishop, ed. 1991. *Being deaf: The experience of deafness.* London: Pinter.

Taylor, G., and A. Darby, ed. 2003. *Deaf identities.* Coleford, United Kingdom: Douglas McLean.

Tsavdaridis, N., and B. Hailstone. 2002. Ethical storm rages over defiant lesbian couple's decision: Disabled baby boy a wish come true. *Adelaide Advertiser,* April 13, 34.

U.S. Food and Drug Administration (U.S. FDA). 2002/2003. *FDA public health web notification: Risk of bacterial meningitis in children with cochlear implants.* Updated September 25, 2003, from original publication, July 24, 2002. http://www.fda.gov/cdrh/safety/cochlear.html.

United Nations Educational, Scientific and Cultural Organization (UNESCO). 2002. *World Conference on Science: Key documents.* http://www.unesco.org/science/wcs/eng/key_documents.htm.

University of Michigan. 2005. U-M scientists develop first micro-machined mechanical cochlea. *News Service,* February 2, n.p. http://www.umich.edu/news/index.html?Releases/2005/Feb05/r020205b.

Walz, C. 2005. Army, navy share specialties for patients' sake. *The Journal,* February 10. http://www.dcmilitary.com/dcmilitary_archives/stories/021005/33280-1.shtml

Welsh, C. n.d. *International documents in support of claims of the existence of electromagnetic anti-personnel weapons.* http://www.mindjustice.org/9.htm.

Wrigley, O. 1996. *The Politics of deafness.* Washington, D.C.: Gallaudet University Press.

2

CONSENT TO SURGERY FOR DEAF CHILDREN: MAKING INFORMED DECISIONS

Priscilla Alderson

This chapter reviews the background social and ethical debates as well as the decision-making frameworks that are concerned with surgery for children. When choices are very hard to make and when the outcomes and balance of potential harms and benefits are complicated or disputed or uncertain, then it can be helpful to follow the processes of making the decision extremely carefully. Even if the decision that is eventually made turns out to be unfortunate, its outcome may be easier to bear if the people concerned can believe that they made the decision in the most informed and committed way that they could and that they knowingly undertook the risks. This chapter, therefore, reviews ethical debates and frameworks as well as questions for decision making that people who are considering surgery such as cochlear implants may wish to consider. The chapter is written ostensibly for responsible adults, although many points also concern children who are able to share in making decisions, and it reviews ways of assessing children's competence to consent.

BACKGROUND SOCIAL DEBATES AND QUESTIONS

Modern societies exert many pressures on their members to treat the body as an unfinished project that should be maintained in a healthy and attractive state. The beauty and keep-fit industries are now complemented by the growing plastic surgery business. The use of technologies from make up to slimming aids to hip replacements is seen as responsible, socially advantageous, and (by some people) moral and almost obligatory. Although cochlear implants are not cosmetic, they are part of the powerful current trends to use technical aids to alter, adapt, and "improve" the natural body. The trends confirm the dominant view that deafness is an impairment, which therefore requires treatments to restore or confer normality. In contrast, the Deaf society argues that deafness can be part of the range of normality and that surgery such as cochlear implants is therefore not only unnecessary but also harmful. When considering a cochlear implant, informed decision making involves questioning these trends reflectively and asking Whom do they really benefit? Are such aids as essential and beneficial as is usually claimed? If the trends are taken for granted, then people are liable to opt for the treatment in question, believing TINA (There Is No Alternative), an assumption that prevents one from thinking critically and making wise choices.

Through people's extensive use of body improvers, notions of an authentic self or identity are blurring into concepts of expressing and fulfilling the self through adopting changing fashions and bodily appearances. The fulfillment partly comes through the perceived or actual social and economic advantages that a "better" looking and functioning body might bring. One great difference between adults and young children is that, however much they are pressured by fashion or peers or employers, adults usually have some choice in whether they alter their body, particularly if they must decide about something as serious as surgery. Young children, however, may not be informed or offered choices about preserving or altering their identity.

"Preserving identity" might even seem to be an irrelevant concept for young children. They may be seen as not yet having any identity to alter, or at least not yet a fixed identity. Rather, their selfhood tends to be seen as fluid, developing, growing, and changing toward adult maturity, and adults must help children and choose for them in this process. The history of childhood is much concerned with adults' efforts to shape children socially, emotionally, educationally, and physically. The term *orthopedics* literally means correcting children. The greater the adults' conviction that this shaping effort is for the child's own good, the less likely they are to doubt their decisions or to consult the child. Parenting is inevitably very much concerned, whether it is willing and conscious or not, with shaping or influencing children. However, rapid changes in childrearing trends leave each generation critical and sometimes shocked about past practices (Hardyment 1984; Miller 1985; Cooter 1992). These ever changing practices remind us how vital it is for parents to ask, Am I really doing this for my child's sake or because of experts' advice or to avoid being criticized?

The past century has seen a great increase in pressure on parents from expert practitioners, politicians, advertisers, and journalists who compel them to micromanage their children (Rose 1990; Hendrick 2003). Yet parents also have to encourage their children to be flourishing individual, independent people. Today's idea of personal identity is that of everyone partly shaping his or her own identity. Bauman (1999, 21) considers "protean being" and endless opportunities, and analyzes both the profound insecurity such fluid identity involves and the complications of trying to be individual and yet accepted. Similarly, Kittay (2006) reflects on the paradox of the desire to be both different and normal. When parents relate to their child as a person rather than as a project, they learn from their child how children achieve their sense of identity. Mayall (1993) noted this difference between parents' and practitioners' attitudes when she interviewed the mothers of twenty-month-old children and their health visitors (community nurses who promote family health). The health visitors, even those who were mothers, were guided by textbooks on how to discipline and stimulate the children. If there were a family party, for example, health visitors would advise that the children must go to bed at their correct time and that mothers should control and stimulate their child as a kind of work project. The mothers saw their children as people, important members of the family party, negotiating rules and stimulating their mothers rather than needing adult stimulation.

This example challenges dominant assumptions that young children are somehow mindless, wholly dependent puppets who are not yet people with their own views and values. In many ways, young children are agents and contributors who dynamically influence their family through imaginative initiatives and through expressions of love, joy, fear, anger, and excitement, often skillfully obtaining what they want through protests, persuasion, and charm (Dunn 1988; Alderson 2001). When children are respected as people in their own right, the questions for the caring adults reflect that respect: Would I want to be treated in the way I am treating my child? And even if I personally prefer my decision, would my child understand and prefer it, both now and in years to come? No two people necessarily share the same views, and a hearing parent and a deaf child may form very different values at some stage.

Among the differences between many able and many disabled people are beliefs in powerful scripts that form our values and decision making. The scripts include triumph and tragic stories, medical and social models of disability, "being normal" and therefore "being abnormal." Oliver (1996), Corker (1998), and others (see Ladd, this volume) have criticized the "triumph or tragedy" accounts that personalize and depoliticize disability. Parents who did not know much about disability before the birth of their impaired child are likely to meet practitioners who tell them, impairment is a tragedy, but with our help you can triumph over your personal difficulties to a great extent. Many disabled people reply, How exactly is it a tragedy? And if we rely on medical remedies, which may carry more costs than benefits, might we reinforce the main problems of social attitudes of stigma or pity and the assumption that it is unbearable to live with the untreated impairment? The history of signing, a communication mode that teachers and doctors tried to stop in the past, warns against placing undue faith in contemporary proposed alternatives to deaf people's chosen ways to communicate. Some doctors have serious reservations that a cochlear implant that is inserted into too young a child may prevent the layer of cells needed to hear from developing (personal communication, Kristen Gerencher, May 20, 2004), although as more effective cochlear implants are gradually developed, the ethical cost-benefits considerations alter.

The question How exactly is deafness a tragedy? leads us to examine the social and medical models of disability. The medical model regards atypical bodies as having illness or injury that must be cured, if possible, or at least managed medically. The fault lies in the child, and the child can come to be defined in the medical view by the condition, by loss or deficiency, thereby ignoring many other aspects of the child's identity, relationships, and daily life. That attitude not only can increase the assumed effects of conditions such as deafness but also tends to foster fears and hopeless myths about the condition. Hearing parents may then feel more anxious and dependent on medical solutions.

Habermas (1979, discussed in Scambler 1987) sees the "life-world" of human agency and communication that enables implicit social integration and personality to be colonized by the "system" of explicit formal, rational state economics and by technology that reduces social questions about how to live with an impairment to technical ones about how to fix it. The value attributed to science overtakes other values, preventing the life-world and the system from being in balance. In some ways, the cost-benefit technical arguments to support cochlear implants contrast with the life-world arguments of the Deaf community. The way that "system" values dominate the debate is illustrated in countless examples, and just one instance is the BBC *News Health* headline (April 28, 2004) previewing an article in the June 2004 issue of *American Journal of Human Genetics*: "Signing 'Increases Deafness Rates.'" The news item reports how signing encourages deaf people to meet and to marry and have children, events that the life-world might celebrate rather than implicitly deplore in the way the news item does.

The social model regards conditions such as being profoundly deaf as compatible with a fulfilled life. Faults or obstacles lie in uncaring societies that refuse to promote inclusive attitudes and environments. The two models—the medical model and the social model—have been theorized by disabled academics and activists. Children, too, can arrive at profound understandings through their hard-won experiential knowledge, as shown by some of the disabled children I have interviewed about their consent to surgery (Alderson 1993). For example, Tina, at age 12, resisted attempts to increase her short stature. She wanted people to accept her as she was, and she could not see why she should adapt for their sake.

In our research about special education (Alderson and Goodey 1998), we found that inclusive education depends on policy changes. One education authority had closed its special schools and had transferred the resources, expertise, and funding into mainstream schools so that most children now attend their nearest school. In that area, deaf children attend dedicated mainstream schools where groups of deaf children can enjoy one another's company and also friendships with hearing children. Everyone in the school learns British Sign Language to some extent. Within this education service that practices the social model of disability, the staff members work out the particular needs of each child as educational concerns rather than medical or psychological concerns, and they also promote activities that everyone can enjoy. They believe that their attention to different needs tends to benefit all children whatever their age, socioeconomic and ethnic background, first language, or ability.

The script about "being normal" is told in different ways. Parents tend to want to help their child to be "normal" enough to be easily accepted and included so that the children are liked and loved and feel at ease with themselves as well as with other people. And yet, as Kittay (2006) considers, who wants their children to be so "normal" that they have no distinctive features or notable idiosyncrasies? Normal can be boringly bland. In contrast, variety may be valued. Yet how different or unusual does a child have to be before that variation counts as unacceptably outside the "normal" range? The accepted range depends on values and attitudes rather than on the child's abilities. In segregated communities, "normal" can have quite narrow meanings of "like us and not like them, the others." This meaning can heighten the anxiety of everyone who is or might be borderline or excluded. In inclusive communities, "normal" has far broader meanings so that, for example, children who use wheelchairs or who have learning difficulties refer to themselves, when talking with others, as normal and consider that they live ordinary, average lives (Alderson and Goodey 1998). Similarly, Deaf communities consider that they and their lifestyles are normal, a word that denies personal tragedy or triumph, though it can involve campaigning to be included in better designed and organized communities.

Bioethics, Values, and Rights

This chapter on consent has discussed the social background for three reasons. First, the threads of these social questions run through all decisions about treatment for disability whether they are recognized or not. Second, early on and often before they realize, parents begin to make choices: trying to adapt the child to fit society's demands or trying to adapt their society and community to fit their child, emphasizing either the medical or the social model, treating their child primarily as a person with an identifiable identity or as a project. Many people avoid these rather starkly expressed choices and try to combine the opposing pairs. However, their first choices or emphases are likely to guide their later decisions, such as a decision to consent to cochlear implant. Any discussion of that decision, which does not first look at the prior background values, effectively narrows the potential options and restricts how critically they can all be scrutinized. The third reason for attending to the social context is that the bioethics literature on consent tends to ignore these background social values and the politics of disability, thereby tending to adopt the medical model. Bioethics also, I suggest, is stacked against disability and assumes narrow concepts of desirable normality. For example, several bioethicists have been saying for years that they favor infanticide of impaired babies (Kuhse and Singer 1985; Harris 1990). These bioethicists appear to hold not only very low expectations of the quality of life of disabled babies and children but also very high expectations of what a minimally tolerable life will be. Inevitably, they then tend to conclude that death is preferable to a disabled life, and they see babies less as persons with identities than as projects to satisfy their parents' preferences.

For example, Caplan (1999, 2000), an official bioethics adviser to the U.S. human genome program, advocates moving on from correcting impairments to enhancing children's appearance or abilities. He predicts that doctors will routinely make total DNA scans, advise on healthy lifestyles, as well as select and enhance embryos. Routine brain scans will enable doctors to control behaviors and learning difficulties and employers to select new staff members. "The rush to use eugenics will be amazing with parents competing to give their kids the best start in life. Many parents will leap at the chance to make their children smarter, fitter and prettier" (Caplan 1999, n.p.). Caplan (2000, n.p.) continues that "technology that simply makes for better children" will overtake ethical concerns. "In a competitive market society, people are going to want to give their kids an edge. . . . [A] genetic edge is not greatly different from an environmental edge. . . . You might download French into the 3-year-old's brain directly." And Murray (2005), anticipates: "Eugenics, anathema today, will be a spin off of the neurogenetic revolution tomorrow. . . . [S]ome parents will, if they can, opt to make their babies more compassionate, or more competitive [mainly] to avoid birth defects [and to choose] improved overall physical and mental abilities. I find it hard to get upset about that prospect".

The quoted examples from Caplan (1999, 2000) were certainly not given to suggest that choosing to insert a cochlear implant is like choosing to make a child "smarter and prettier." The cochlear implant decision is about trying to correct or relieve an impairment whereas the futuristic genetic choices are about trying to increase or enhance a child's characteristics, striving for the "supernormal." The point of the examples is to illustrate the very different types of values on which the social or the medical models of disability are based, although the social model does accept that medical aid can uniquely remedy certain illnesses. The challenge for parents and patients is to decide when medical treatment really is the best remedy for a problem and when other remedies, social or political ones, may be more effective, for example, better education and employment systems.

The idea of treating the child as a project rather than as a person resonates with fairly widespread views, and parents may expect this approach to be one reward for having children. For example, Ross, a pediatrician, proposes that "for many adults, rearing a child in an environment in which their [the parents'] values and beliefs flourish is a principal reason for becoming a parent" (Ross 1998, 6). Although this observation is partly true, it can become a dangerous and oppressive desire. How can parents such as these cope when their children adopt other values and beliefs, as they are highly likely to do? Is it healthy to strive to produce children who are in effect moral and social clones of the parents? And would not parents and children be happier if the parents' values were to include tolerance of difference and respect for diversity?

Edwards (2006) warns that technology is not morally neutral, and he draws on Heidegger's (1977) work to reflect on how technology alters how we regard and relate to things. We come to see things as *Bestand*, a standing reserve for our use. A forest, for example, becomes a source of wood and paper to serve our wants. "Everywhere, everything is ordered to stand by, to be immediately on hand, indeed to stand there just so that it may be a call for further ordering" (Heidegger cited in Edwards 2006, 52). The greater danger is that we come to see other people, particularly children, as a standing reserve ready to meet our needs and desires. Edwards (58) asks, "Are we (with the best of intentions, of course) treating the child's body (and life) as *Bestand*, as raw material to be shaped so as to fit our (and presumably [the child's]) sense of what is 'natural,' 'normal' and 'orderly'? And if we are, is anything wrong with that?" Efforts to avoid following fashions and seemingly indubitable common sense can involve asking hard and unusual questions such as Why do I want my child to be normal? and What does normal mean?

James Edwards belonged to a working group that produced the book *Surgically Shaping Children* (Parens 2006). Another member of the group, Cassandra Aspinell, was born with a cleft lip and palate. She has a son with this condition, and she is a social worker in a cleft surgical team. Her chapter "Do I Make You Uncomfortable?" (Aspinell 2006) warns parents who choose corrective surgery in the belief that it demonstrates their love and concern for their child. The child may perceive that what underlies the choice and the parents' desire to help the child to be socially accepted is a rejection of the child's original and "real" identity. In this paradox, the child may experience the parents' gesture of love in the opposite way to what was intended.

A positive and mutually respectful basis for relationships between parents and children is advocated in the United Nations (UN) Convention on the Rights of the Child (UN 1989). The Convention accepts that children need loving families, although love cannot be a right, and it sets out many ways for states to support and nurture families. The Convention also (a) respects children's rights to "preserve [their] identity . . . without unlawful interference" (Article 8), (b) advocates for due account to be taken of their views as soon as they are able to form and express views (Article 12), and (c) affirms disabled children's rights to "enjoy a full and decent life, in conditions that ensure dignity, promote self-reliance and facilitate the child's active participation in the community" (Article 23). The Convention is not prescriptive. Instead of providing simple answers, it offers guiding principles to help people who are trying to make the best or least harmful decisions for and with children.

Bioethics is often advanced as a neutral method for reaching the best decision. Yet underlying the bioethicists' predictions are leading principles that can be interpreted in hostile ways toward disabled people. The principles are autonomy, justice, and nonmaleficence (Beauchamp and Childress 2000). Concepts of autonomy highly value independent, intelligent adults and so implicitly accord less value to people with learning difficulties and those who are emotionally or economically dependent, the inevitable state of early childhood. The cool idealizing of implicitly lonely autonomy ignores how we are all interdependent and how we can be enriched rather than simply constricted by close personal ties and obligations. Justice, in the social model of disability, concerns changing society to respect rights and to increase inclusion, equality, and the just redistribution of resources. However, bioethicists tend to interpret justice as keeping the rules of the status quo and present inequality, for example, by avoiding taxation and emphasizing rationed, targeted use of resources. Nonmaleficence, or do no harm, is often debated in a curiously disembodied way, with concern to avoid intrusion or disrespect. These are important concerns, but the notion of harm loses much of its meaning unless ethicists take embodied, emotional and social suffering seriously.

However, autonomy, justice, and do no harm can be valuable principles for thinking about cochlear implants. Might the whole procedure enhance the child's autonomy, sensory experiences, relationships, thoughts, and feelings? Alternatively, might her autonomy best be respected by accepting her present identity and concentrating on adapting her circumstances to help her to have rich experiences and a fulfilled personal and social life? Is the justice of equal opportunities and of fair distribution and enjoyment of resources best served by providing the surgery or by alternative methods? And would the child feel most harmed by being deprived of the opportunity of surgery or by having it, in a sense, imposed? How successful is the procedure likely to be? And how is success defined and measured, for example, in terms of hearing acuity, language, communication and academic skills, social relationships, or reported satisfactions? How much time and effort are required to help the child to learn to use the implant compared with the effort required to learn without the implant? Might the implant preclude the hope of using better technology if that technology were developed in the future? Is responsibility being transferred on to the child to adapt to a hearing world and to save her family and friends from adapting and learning to sign and to use other communication? Might the child prefer to be bilingual and use signing and speech?

Davis (2001) carefully reviews the pros and cons of cochlear implants, but then draws her own conclusion in favor of them, arguing that the child has the right to an open future and therefore ought to have the chances the implant might offer. One difficulty here is the suggestion that there is a correct decision or solution; some parents, however, may be equally convinced by the opposite view.

A second difficulty is the concept of an open future and the idea that childhood ought to be malleable, lacking fixed identity, without allowing time to leave doors open and to venture far in any direction that might close off other options. However, an insistence on childhood "openness" inevitably closes off commitments that children may want to make, identities they may wish to adopt. It also denies that all through our lives we leave some options open, close others, and sometimes reopen them. In contrast, Mary John (2003) is committed to respecting children's rights, their knowledge, power, and agency now, and she traces her conviction back to her wounding, solitary experiences in hospital when she was the age of seven years and, for weeks, had no visitors and no explanations.

Competent Children

There are four levels of involving children in making decisions: to inform them, to listen to their views, to take due account of their informed views, and to respect the child as the decision maker (Alderson and Montgomery 1996). The Convention on the Rights of the Child (UN 1989) respects children's rights to form and express views as soon as they are able to do so. English law, which influences laws in Commonwealth countries, goes further and respects children's own decisions as long as the child is deemed to be competent (see *Gillick v. Wisbech and W. Norfolk HA* [1985] 3 All ER 423). Neither *Gillick* nor the Convention states an age when competence begins. Competence entails understanding the relevant issues; being able to weigh them and to make an informed choice; and in the case of decisions about interventions on children, respecting the child's welfare and best interests (*Gillick v. Wisbech and W. Norfolk HA*). Competence also involves the autonomy to have the courage and resolve to make an emotionally as well as intellectually difficult decision and to stand by it however risky and even mistaken it may turn out to be.

There are three ways to assess whether a child is competent (Brazier and Lobjoit 1991). The first involves assessing the child's status, including age (but English law does not support this approach for decisions about health care). The second involves assessing outcome, or quality of the decision made (which can unfairly depend on whether the assessor happens to agree with it or not). The third involves assessing the process of decision making and whether it was well reasoned. The third method is the fairest way and can include checking whether the child understands the nature and purpose of the intervention, the risks and hoped for benefits, and the alternatives.

However, besides assessing the child, it is also important to assess the adults concerned. Have they informed the child clearly, fully, and honestly? Do they trust and respect the child's autonomy and courage to know and undertake the risks? Are they willing to understand the child's views as reasonable, even if they disagree with them? It seems that children and adults rarely disagree over major treatment, and if they do, there tends also to be disagreement among the adults about determining the best course. In cases of uncertainty, arguably it is even more important to listen and, when possible, to involve the child in decision making (Alderson 1993; Parens 2006). The person who lives in, and is, the body being considered for surgery has unique and essential knowledge about his or her best interests. From a early age, children begin to hold values and preferences, although for people of any age these are influenced by their family, friends, the mass media, literature, and many other factors. Children vary greatly in how able and willing they are to share in or to make hard choices, so adults need to be sensitive to children's cues and preferences.

Two Kinds of Bioethics

Frank (2006) identifies two contrasting forms of bioethics: protectionist and Socratic. Along with principles and analytical debates, protectionist bioethics has clarified the elements of informed consent in valuable, protective ways (*Nuremberg Code* 1947; WMA 1964/2000). Consent is informed when the people concerned understand in detail the purpose and nature of the procedure and what is entailed, the short-term and longer term effects, the likely risks, the hoped for benefits, and any alternatives. Consent is voluntary when it is not hurried or pressured, when people have time to evaluate the information and arrive at a freely made decision. There should be no force or deceit or pressure. Parents will feel pressured by their child's needs, but they should not be pressured or persuaded by the clinical staff. People should also be aware that consent is a choice to say either yes or no; they often assume they have to agree. They should be told that they have time to consider and to ask questions and, perhaps, to negotiate aspects of the decision such as the timing. Although some bioethicists say that there should be no pressures at all on the person's autonomous decision, others argue that without numerous social influences as well as formative experiences and values, we would have no choices, so autonomy therefore entails being as aware as possible of the salient factors and their background, which the first section of this chapter has partly reviewed.

Doctors strive to draw their information from evidence-based medicine, the evidence ideally being derived from randomized controlled trials (RCTs), the "gold standard" and a uniquely rigorous research method for testing whether treatments are helpful, harmful, or ineffective. However, RCTs are complicated and expensive, and so far, they have tested relatively few treatments. The results of many RCTs have not been reported. Some RCTs are funded by the firms that produce the medicines or equipment being assessed, so there may be pressure on researchers to overreport benefits and underreport harms. When the full effects of treatment are not known for five, ten, or more years later and if they test past treatments that have been replaced by newer ones, then the results of the RCT will be out of date before they are reported. It is easier to test the clinical effects of a treatment than to test the social effects, and it is easier to prove, for example, that a drug has cured a disease than to demonstrate how people live happier more fulfilled lives because they have a cochlear implant. Influenced by the medical model of disability, clinical RCTs are limited in how they can design and compare social interventions with medical ones, for example, comparing the effects of providing either cochlear implant surgery or else psychosocial and educational support and changed social policies for deaf children.

Doctors who conduct trials should have equipoise; that is, they should sincerely believe that each of the two or more treatments being tested offers the child an equal chance of benefit and risk of harm. They should at least believe that, despite their personal view, the relative harms and benefits are so unknown that it is ethical to enter a child for any of the interventions in the trial. Yet it may be hard to find enough doctors who believe that it is ethical not to provide cochlear implants. For these reasons, doctors cannot fully inform parents about the risks and benefits of cochlear implants.

Although protectionist bioethics and its analysis of informed and voluntary consent is very practical and useful, Frank (2006) views it as limited and mainly concerned with costs and risks and with the protecting of practitioners from blame if harm occurs. Frank describes a contrasting Socratic ethics, concerned with deep questions such as What is the good life? What kind of life do I want to live? What kind of person do I want to be? And what kinds of communities do I want to live in? For potentially irrevocable life-changing procedures such as the cochlear implant, these questions are vital ones to ask, especially when parents are deciding on their child's behalf. The questions may initiate a journey of discovery about hearing and deaf individuals and communities, which will perhaps enrich the life of the child and family, whatever choice the parents take. The Socratic questions enlarge attention beyond the individual child and family toward the potential collective effects of personal decisions. How might attitudes and relationships between hearing and deaf people be affected by the individual decision in ways that either open or close mutual respect and understanding? These general matters are likely to affect the child's future.

This discussion ends with questions posed by Winkler (1998, 249) to help people who are reflecting on whether to accept a treatment. Does it "enhance the whole person or offer only a palliative substitute for wholeness? Does it serve our desires for completeness and connection, or pander to our anxieties and our short-sighted demands for control? Finally, does the technology and its application help us to love and honor the body in all its fragility, imperfection and finitude?"

References

Alderson, P. 1993. *Children's consent to surgery.* Buckingham, United Kingdom: Open University Press.

———. 2001. Life and death: Agency and dependency in young children's health care. *Children'z Issues* 5 (1):23–7.

Alderson, P., and C. Goodey. 1998. *Enabling education: Experiences in special and ordinary schools.* London: Tufnell Press.

Alderson, P., and J. Montgomery. 1996. *Health care choices: Making decisions with children.* London: Institute for Public Policy Research.

Aspinell, C. 2006. "Do I make you uncomfortable?" Reflections on using surgery to reduce the distress of others. In *Surgically shaping children: Technology, ethics, and the pursuit of normality,* ed. E. Parens, 13–28. Baltimore: Johns Hopkins University Press.

Bauman, Z. 1999. *In search of politics.* Cambridge, United Kingdom: Polity Press.

Beauchamp, T., and J. Childress. 2000. *Principles of biomedical ethics.* New York: Oxford University Press.

Brazier, M., and M. Lobjoit, ed. 1991. *Protecting the vulnerable: Autonomy and consent in health care.* London: Routledge.

Caplan, A. 1999. Bioethics 100 years from now. *Techno-Eugenics News* 1 (October 9).

Cooter, R. 1992. *In the name of the child: Health and welfare 1880–1940.* London: Routledge.

Corker, M. 1998. *Deaf and disabled? Or deafness disabled.* Buckingham: Open University Press.

Davis, D. 2001. *Genetic dilemmas: Reproductive technology, parental choices, and children's futures.* New York: Routledge.

Dunn, J. 1988. *The beginnings of social understanding.* Oxford, United Kingdom: Blackwell.

Edwards, J. 2006. Concepts of technology and their role in moral reflection. In *Surgically shaping children: Technology, ethics, and the pursuit of normality,* ed. E. Parens, 51–67. Baltimore: Johns Hopkins University Press.

Frank, A. 2006. Emily's scars: Surgical shapings, technolux, and bioethics. In *Surgically shaping children: Technology, ethics, and the pursuit of normality,* ed. E. Parens, 68–89. Baltimore: Johns Hopkins University Press.

Gerencher, K. 2004. Practical genomics: Genetic testing to tailor health care. *Human Genetics Alert News,* May 20. http://www.nga.org.uk.

Habermas, J. 1979. *Communication and the evolution of society.* London: Heinemann.

Hardyment, C. 1984. *Dream babies: Child care from Locke to Spock.* Oxford: Oxford University Press.

Harris, J. 1990. Wrongful birth. In *Philosophical ethics in reproductive medicine,* ed. D. Bromham, M. Dalton, and J. Jackson, 156–70. Manchester, United Kingdom: Manchester University Press.

Heidegger, M. 1977. *Basic writing.* Edited by D. Krell. New York: Harper and Row.

Hendrick, H. 2003. *Child welfare: Historical dimensions, contemporary debate.* Bristol: Policy Press.

John, M. 2003. *Children's rights and power.* London: Jessica Kingsley.

Kittay, E. 2006. Thoughts on the desire for normality. In *Surgically shaping children: Technology, ethics, and the pursuit of normality,* ed. E. Parens, 90–112. Baltimore: Johns Hopkins University Press.

Kuhse, H., and P. Singer. 1985. *Should the baby live?* Oxford: Oxford University Press.

Mayall, B. 1993. Keeping children healthy. *Social Science and Medicine* 36: 77–84.

Miller, A. 1985. *Thou shalt not be aware: Society's betrayal of the child.* London: Pluto Press.

Murray, C. 2005. Deeper into the brain. *U.S. National Review,* January 24.

Nuremberg Code. 1947. http://ohsr.od.nih.gov/guidelines/nuremberg.html.

Oliver, M. 1996. *Understanding disability: From theory to practice.* Basingstoke, United Kingdom: Macmillan.

Parens, E., ed. 2006. *Surgically shaping children: Technology, ethics, and the pursuit of normality.* Baltimore: Johns Hopkins University Press.

Rose, N. 1990. *Governing the soul.* London: Routledge.

Ross, L. F. 1998. *Children, families, and health care decision-making.* Oxford, United Kingdom: Clarendon Press.

Scambler, G. 1987. Habermas and the power of medical expertise. In *Sociological theory and medical sociology,* ed. G. Scambler, 59–73. London: Tavistock.

United Nations (UN). 1989. *Convention on the rights of the child*. Geneva: United Nations.

Winkler, M. 1998. The devices and desires or our own hearts. In *Enhancing human traits: Ethical and social implications*, ed. E. Parens, 238–50. Washington, D.C.: Georgetown University Press.

World Medical Association (WMA). 1964/2000. *Declaration of Helsinki*. Fernay-Voltaire, France: WMA.

3
ETHNICITY, ETHICS, AND THE DEAF-WORLD

Harlan Lane

This chapter is concerned with ethical aspects of the relationships among language minorities using signed languages (called the Deaf-World) and the larger societies that engulf them. It undertakes to show that such minorities have the properties of ethnic groups and that an unsuitable construction of the Deaf-World as a disability group has led to programs of the majority that not only discourage Deaf children from acquiring the language and culture of the Deaf-World but also intend to reduce the number of Deaf births—programs that are unethical from an ethnic-group perspective. The chapter advances four reasons not to construe the Deaf-World as a disability group: (1) Deaf people themselves do not believe they have a disability; (2) the disability construction brings with it needless medical and surgical risks for the Deaf child; (3) the disability construction also endangers the future of the Deaf-World; and finally, (4) the disability construction brings bad solutions to real problems because it is predicated on a misunderstanding.

It has become widely known that, as in other nations, there is a Deaf-World in the United States that comprises citizens whose primary language is American Sign Language and who identify as members of that minority culture. The size of the population is not known, but estimates generally range from half a million to a million members (Schein 1989). The English terms *deaf* and *hearing impaired* are commonly used to designate a much larger and more heterogeneous group than the members of the Deaf-World. Most of the 20 million Americans (Binnie 1994) who are in that larger group had conventional schooling and became deaf after acculturation to hearing society; they communicate primarily in English or one of the spoken minority languages; they generally do not have Deaf spouses; they do not identify themselves as members of the Deaf-World, nor do they use its language, participate in its organizations, profess its values, or behave in accord with its mores; rather, they consider themselves hearing people with a disability. Something similar is true of most nations: there is a Deaf-World, a relatively small group of visual people (Bahan 2005; Padden and Humphries 1988) who use a natural visual-gestural language and who are often confused with the larger group of people who view themselves as hearing impaired and who use a spoken language in its spoken or written form. Acknowledgment of this contrast, often signaled in the scholarly literature by the use of capital-D *Deaf* for members of the Deaf-World and small-d *deaf* for members of the larger group, does not deny that there is a gray area between the two groups; for example, some hard of hearing people are active in the American Deaf-World while others are not. Oral deaf adults and late-deafened adults usually consider that they have a hearing impairment and do not self-identify as members of the Deaf-World.

This chapter is concerned exclusively with the smaller group, the Deaf-World. The discussion undertakes to show that it qualifies as an ethnic group and that an unsuitable construction of the Deaf-World as a disability group has led to programs (such as oral education and cochlear implant surgery) that discourage Deaf children from participating in the Deaf-World and that attempt to reduce the number of Deaf births—programs that are unethical from an ethnic-group perspective. In other words, this chapter makes the case that our ethical standards for the majority's treatment of Deaf people depend, not surprisingly, on whether our representation of the Deaf-World is that of a disability group or that of an ethnic group.

The Deaf-World Is an Ethnic Group

A strong case can be made that the Deaf-World is an ethnic group. Support for this case can be found by considering the very criteria and characteristics that social scientists use to characterize any ethnic group: internal properties and ethnic boundaries.

Internal Properties

Table 3.1 shows the criteria that social scientists have advanced for characterizing a social group as an ethnic group.

1. *Collective name.* The members of this group have a collective name in their manual-visual language by which they refer to themselves. I will refer to them by that name in adopting the English translation of their compound sign DEAF-WORLD.

2. *Feeling of community.* Self-recognition, and recognition by others, is a central feature of ethnicity (Barth 1969; Smith 1986). Americans in the Deaf-World do indeed feel a strong identification with that world and show great loyalty to it. This loyalty is not surprising; the Deaf-World offers many Deaf Americans what they could not find at home: easy communication, a positive identity, a surrogate family. The Deaf-World has the highest rate of endogamous members of any ethnic group—an estimated 90 percent (Schein 1989).

3. *Norms for behavior.* In Deaf culture, there are norms for relating to the Deaf-World, including norms for decision making (consensus is the rule, not individual initiative), for managing information, for constructing discourse, for gaining status, for managing indebtedness, and many more. Cultural rules are not honored all the time by everyone any more than are linguistic rules. Such rules tell what you must know as a member of a particular linguistic and cultural group, but what one actually does or says depends on a host of intervening factors, including other rules that have priority.

Table 3.1. Properties of Ethnic Groups: Distinct	
Collective Name	Customs
Feeling of community	Social structure
Norms for behavior	Language
Values	Art Forms
Knowledge	History
	Kinship

4. *Distinct values.* The underlying values of an ethnic group can often be inferred from cultural norms. A value that appears to be fundamental in the Deaf-World is allegiance to the culture, which is expressed in the prizing of one's membership in the Deaf-World, in endogamous marriage, in the gaining of status by enhancing the group and acknowledging its contributions, in the giving of culturally related names, in consensual decision making, in the defining of oneself in relation to the culture, in distributed indebtedness, in the priority given to evidence that arises from experience as a member of the culture, in the treasuring of the language of the Deaf-World, and in efforts among Deaf people to promote the dissemination of culturally salient information (Smith 1997; Mindess 1999; Lane 2004a).

5. *Knowledge.* Deaf people have culture-specific knowledge such as who their leaders are (and what their characteristics are), the concerns of rank-and-file members of the Deaf-World, important events in Deaf history, and how to manage in trying situations with hearing people. Knowing when and with whom to use American Sign Language and when to use English-marked varieties of signed language is an important part of being recognized as Deaf (Johnson and Erting 1989).

6. *Customs.* The Deaf-World has its own ways of doing introductions and departures, of taking turns in a conversation, of speaking frankly, and of speaking politely; it also has its own taboos.

7. *Social structure.* There are numerous organizations in the American Deaf-World, including those that are athletic, social, political, literary, religious, and fraternal (Lane, Hoffmeister, and Bahan 1996). As with many ethnic minorities, there are charismatic leaders who are felt to embody the unique characteristics of the whole ethnic group (Smith 1986).

8. *Language.* Competence in American Sign Language is a hallmark of Deaf ethnicity in the United States and some other parts of North America. A language not based on sound is the primary element that sharply demarcates the Deaf-World from the engulfing hearing society.

> The mother tongue is an aspect of the soul of a people. It is their achievement par excellence. Language is the surest way for individuals to safeguard or recover the authenticity they inherited from their ancestors as well as to hand it on to generations yet unborn. (Fishman 1989, 276)

9. *The arts.* Consider first the language arts through which the Deaf-World expresses itself. There are narratives in American Sign Language (ASL), storytelling, oratory, humor, tall tales, word play, pantomime, and poetry. Theatre arts and the visual arts also address Deaf culture and experience.

10. *History.* Ethnic groups construct rootedness, whose forms of expression include history, territory, and genealogy. The Deaf-World has a rich history recounted in stories, books, films, and the like. Members of the Deaf-World have a particular interest in their history because "the past is a resource in the collective quest for meaning [and ethnic identity]" (Nagel 1994, 163). A sense of common history unites successive generations (Fishman 1982, 1989; Smith, 1986).

11. *Kinship.* Many ethnic groups have a belief in the land of their ancestors. However, "territory is relevant not because it is actually possessed but because of an alleged and felt connection. The land of dreams is far more significant than any actual terrain" (Smith 1986, 34). Land that the Deaf-World in the United States has traditionally felt an attachment to includes the residential schools; Deaf travel is often planned around visits to some of those schools. There is a Deaf utopian vision of "a land of our own" expressed in folk tales, novels, journalism, theater, and political discussions (Lane 1984; Bullard 1986; Winzer 1986; Van Cleve and Crouch 1989; Levesque 1994). Deaf-Worlds are to be found around the globe, and when Deaf members from two different cultures meet, they feel a strong bond although they share no common territory and are limited in their ability to communicate with one another. In this way, they are like diaspora groups such as the Jews. And like the diaspora ethnic minorities worldwide, prejudice and discrimination in the host society encourage them to cultivate their ethnicity to maintain their dignity despite social marginalization.

Some scholars maintain that the core of ethnicity lies in the cultural properties I have examined, so kinship is not necessary for the Deaf-World or any other group to qualify as an ethnic group (Barth 1969; Schneider 1972; Peterson 1980; Sollors 2001). Others say kinship should be taken in its social meaning as *those to whom we owe primary solidarity* (Schneider 1969). "Ethnie embody the sense of being a large unique family; the members feel knit to one another and so committed to the cultural heritage, which is the family's inheritance" (Smith 1986, 49). What is involved is a sense of tribal belonging, not necessarily genetic and blood ties. Certainly, there is a strong sense of solidarity in the Deaf-World; the metaphor of family goes far in characterizing many Deaf-World norms and practices.

What kinship is really about, other scholars contend, is a link to the past; it is about *intergenerational continuity* (Fishman 1989). The Deaf-World does pass its norms, knowledge, language, and values from one generation to the next: first, through socialization of the child by Deaf adults (parent or other) and, second, through peer socialization. Here, however, there is a significant difference from other ethnic groups: for many Deaf children, socialization into Deaf culture starts late, usually when the Deaf child meets other Deaf children in school (Johnson and Erting 1989).

Members of the Deaf-World have a great handicap and a great advantage when it comes to intergenerational continuity. The handicap is that their hearing parents usually have a different ethnocultural identity that they cannot pass on to their children because a shared language is lacking. Moreover, these hearing parents commonly do not advocate in the schools, community, courts, and so on for their Deaf child's primary language. Minority languages that do not have parental and community support are normally endangered. The great advantage of the Deaf-World lies in the fact that there will always be intergenerational continuity for signed language because there will always be visual people who take possession of that language in preference to any other and with it the wisdom and values of generations of Deaf people before them. (Although one can imagine an intervention in the future that would provide high-fidelity hearing to Deaf children and thus threaten intergenerational continuity, most countries likely would not be able to afford it and most Deaf parents likely would continue to refuse such interventions with their Deaf children.)

When we think of kinship, yet other scholars maintain, the issue is one of common ancestors, what Joshua Fishman (1977) termed "paternity"—real or putative biological connections across generations. Johnson and Erting (1989) suggest that what is primary in this biological criterion for kinship is not genealogy but biological resemblance across generations. In that case, members of the Deaf-World are kin because Deaf people resemble one another biologically in their reliance on vision for language and for much else (Johnson and Erting 1989). To some extent, like the members of many other ethnic groups, Deaf people more often than not come by their biological resemblance through heredity. The estimate commonly cited is 50 to 60 percent of all people born deaf, with little or no usable hearing, are so for hereditary reasons (Reardon et al. 1992). However, another 20 percent are Deaf for reasons unknown; many of those may be hereditarily Deaf people not aware of the role of their ancestry (Smith 1995).

Summarizing the internal properties of ethnic groups in the words of social scientist Arthur Smith,

> By involving a collective name, by the use of symbolic images of community, by the generation of stereotypes of the community and its foes, by the ritual performance and rehearsal of ceremonies, by the communal recitation of past deeds and ancient hero's exploits, men and women partake of a collectivity and its historic fate which transcend their individual existences (Smith 1986, 46).

Many scholars in the field of ethnicity believe that these "internal" properties of the ethnic group just reviewed must also be accompanied by an "external" property, a boundary separating the minority from other ethnicities, in particular, the majority ethnicity (Barth 1969). Does the Deaf-World in the United States occupy its own ecological niche? Does it look to itself for the satisfaction of certain needs while looking to the larger society for the satisfaction of other needs?

Ethnic Boundaries

The left column of table 3.2 shows activities that are primarily conducted by Deaf people for Deaf people in the Deaf-World in the United States; the right column, activities in the hearing world that affect Deaf people; and the middle column, areas of overlap. The more Deaf people celebrate their language and culture, the more they affirm their distinct identity, the more they reinforce the boundary delineating them from the hearing world. Language comes first because it always plays a powerful role in maintaining ethnic boundaries, but it is especially powerful in the case of Deaf people because hearing people are rarely fluent in visual language and members of the Deaf-World are rarely fluent in spoken language. Next, Deaf-World social activities are organized and conducted by Deaf people with little or no involvement from those who are hearing. Law enforcement, however, is a hearing world activity. Religious services overlap the Deaf and hearing worlds; there are missions to the Deaf, Deaf pastors, and signed services, but the operation of the house of worship is generally in hearing hands. All in all, the Deaf-World keeps to itself for many of its activities, it collaborates in a few with the hearing world, and it leaves the really broad responsibilities such as law enforcement to the larger society. In this pattern, it is like other ethnic groups such as Hispanic Americans.

This brief survey is intended to show that the Deaf-World in the United States today meets the criteria put forth for ethnic groups (see also Padden and Markowicz 1976; Erting 1978, 1982; Markowicz and Woodward 1978; Johnson and Erting 1979, 1982, 1984, 1989). Classifying the Deaf-World as an ethnic group should encourage those who are concerned with Deaf people to do appropriate things: learn their language, defend their heritage against more powerful groups, study their ethnic history, and so on. In this light, the Deaf-World should enjoy

Table 3.2. Deaf-World–Hearing World boundaries

Deaf-World	Overlap	Hearing-World
Signed language	Interpreter services	Spoken language
Social activities	Religious services	Law enforcement
Signed language teaching	Consumer goods and services	Employment (not Deaf-related)
Political activities	Deaf history	Military services
Athletics	Deaf education	Garbage collection
Arts and leisure	Deaf service agencies	Medical care
Finding employment		Banking
Publishing		Transportation

the rights and protections accorded other ethnic groups under international law and treaties, including the United Nations' *Declaration on the Rights of Persons Belonging to National or Ethnic, Religious and Linguistic Minorities* (United Nations 1992).

REASONS ADVANCED TO VIEW THE DEAF-WORLD AS A DISABILITY GROUP

Is it appropriate to label the Deaf-World a disability group? We do not ask whether Deaf people in fact have a disability because it is not a matter of fact; disability, like ethnicity, is a social construct, not a fact of life, although one property of such constructs is that they appear misleadingly to be a fact of life. For example, the social problem of alcoholism evidently consists in this: many Americans suffer from the disease of alcoholism, and there are specially trained people to help them—alcoholism counselors, psychologists, psychiatrists and others—and special facilities to care for them such as detox centers. However, this understanding of alcoholism dates from the latter half of the twentieth century. In the first half, the Temperance Movement branded excessive drinking as voluntary, and the movement promoted, not treatment, but prohibition. With the shift in the construction of alcoholism, from illegal (and immoral) behavior to illness, the need also shifted, focusing on medical research and treatment, halfway houses, hospital wards, outpatient clinics, and specialized hospitals (Gusfield 1982).

Homosexuality went from moral flaw, to crime, to treatable disability, to a minority group seeking civil rights (Conrad and Schneider 1980). When growth enzyme was discovered, and not before, shortness came to be seen as a disability of childhood instead of as a normal variation (Werth 1991; Downie et al. 1996). With the arrival of the IQ test, mild mental retardation came to be seen as a disability instead of as merely normal human variation in intellect (Gelb 1987). In societies where signed language use is mostly restricted to Deaf people, hearing people commonly see being Deaf as a serious problem requiring professional intervention, but in societies where signed language use is widespread because of a substantial Deaf population—on Martha's Vineyard and Bali for example—being Deaf is simply seen as a trait, not a disability (Lane, Pillard, and French 2000).

The case of the pygmy forest dwellers of Central Africa is instructive. Their short stature, some four-and-a-half feet on average, allows them modest caloric requirements, easy and rapid passage through dense jungle cover in search of game, and construction of small huts that can be rapidly disassembled and reassembled for self-defense and hunting. The Bantu villagers, formerly herdsmen, now farmers, have contempt for the pygmies because of their puny size, and the pygmies in turn have contempt for the villagers who are "clumsy as elephants" and "do not know how to walk" in the forest, much too tall to move swiftly and silently (Turnbull 1962, 79). Each group considers the other handicapped by the physical size of its members. Each fails to appreciate how physical makeup, culture, and environment are intertwined.

Despite all this evidence that disability is constructed in a given society at a given time, many writers addressing ethics and Deaf people, apparently unaware of disability studies and medical anthropology, simply adopt the naive materialist view when it comes to disability: "Almost by definition deaf persons . . . have a disability" (Gonsoulin 2001, 554); "I maintain that the inability to hear is a deficit, a disability, a lack of perfect health" (Davis 1997, 254). And their ethical conclusions turn on this postulate. We understand, however, that disability is a label that can be applied with more or with less aptness to a particular group. That application is not a matter of chance, even less is it foreordained; it is powerfully influenced by the "technologies of normalization" (Foucault 1980, 21) that exist to mitigate what is seen as a disability, for they have a great stake in retaining that conception of the group. The next section critically examines arguments that have been made for including members of the Deaf-World among disability groups.

Oppression from Deaf Bodies

Those who advocate classifying Deaf people with disability groups claim that Deaf people have something in common with people who avowedly have disabilities: they are discriminated against because general social customs do not accommodate their bodies. Deaf people are indeed discriminated against—in school, on the job, in issues of access, but it is much more their language that is the target of discrimination than their bodies: "the major effect of deafness is on communication" (Baynton 2000, 391). Thus, Deaf groups are more like oppressed language minorities than oppressed disability groups. Like many Hispanic Americans, for example, many Deaf people have difficulty learning in school because the teacher cannot communicate with them fluently; they have difficulty getting a job when the job requires good English; they miss out on important information because it has not been provided in their language.

Still, say the Deaf-are-disabled advocates, why not acknowledge the many things that physically different people share by using a common label (Baynton 2002). After all, some disability activists make a claim for disability culture, just as there is a Deaf culture; many oppose mainstreaming, as do many Deaf activists. Both groups pay the price of social stigma, and stigmatized groups—among them disabled people, blacks, women, gays, and the Deaf—are often claimed to be biologically inferior. Moreover, both the Deaf-World and disability groups struggle with the troubled-persons industries for control of their destiny (Gusfield 1984). Both the Deaf-World and the disability groups endeavor to promote their own construction of their identity in competition with the efforts of professionals to promote *their* constructions. Finally, because there are great differences among disability groups, accommodating one more with its unique issues need not be a problem.

At one level, oppressed minorities do indeed share important traits and a common struggle for the defense and valuing of their diversity. At that level, disabled people, blacks, women, gays, as well as the Deaf and other language minorities can inform and reinforce one another's efforts. They can promote an understanding of the value of diversity, learn successful strategies from one another, and use their combined numbers to urge government in the right directions. At another level, however, many practical truths apply only to individual minorities, each of which has its own make-up, demographics, histories, and cultures. Minimizing that diversity by assigning the same global representation would undermine the most cherished goal of each group—to be respected and valued for its difference. After all, beyond being stigmatized because of their physical difference, what, practically speaking, do the Deaf have in common with gays, women, blacks, Little People, and people with mobility impairment? Deaf people have been subject to the globalizing disability label, and it has widely led to the wrong questions and therefore the wrong answers, which are considered later in this chapter under reasons to reject it. This response is the pragmatic answer to disability scholar Lennard Davis's proposal that Deaf people abandon the category of ethnicity in favor of a coalition with gays, hearing children with Deaf parents, and people with disabilities (Davis 2002): those groups' agendas are utterly different.

The Shared Struggle for Rights

Another argument advanced for having Deaf people embrace the disability label is that it might assist them in gaining more of their rights (Baynton 2002). For example, interpreters are not normally provided in the classroom for members of ethnic groups; Deaf people have them in many places under a disability umbrella. Nevertheless, much that is important to Deaf people has come through an understanding of the Deaf-World as an ethnic group. Consider the burgeoning of ASL in high schools and colleges in the United States and the increasing acceptance of ASL classes in fulfillment of the foreign language and culture requirement; the mushrooming of scholarship in the last forty years concerning Deaf ethnicity—history, arts, social structure, culture, and language; the flourishing of the interpreting profession; the development of the discipline of Deaf Studies; bilingual-bicultural Deaf education; the growing community of nations that formally recognize their national signed language. All these gains reflect an understanding of Deaf people as an ethnic group.

Although the disability label seems inappropriate for the Deaf-World, its members have not aggressively promoted government understanding of its ethnicity and of the poor fit of the disability label. As a result, the majority's accommodation of the Deaf has come under a disability label, and Deaf people must in effect subscribe to that label to gain their rights with respect to information access, education, and other areas. This predicament is the Deaf dilemma: either retain some important rights as members of their society at the expense of being mischaracterized by that society and government or surrender some of those rights in the hope of gradually undermining that misconstruction. This dilemma is reminiscent of similarly oppressive choices offered to other minority groups: to gays—embrace the disability label and you will be spared classification as a criminal and entry into the army; to women—conform to the masculine idea of the feminine ideal and men will support and applaud you.

In principle, it should be possible for members of the Deaf-World in the United States to base their demand for language access on existing legislation and court rulings protecting language minorities. For example, in the field of education, the U.S. Congress has passed two types of statutes to remedy the disadvantage experienced by language-minority students who cannot communicate freely in the classroom by using their primary language. The Bilingual Education Act (Public Law 89-10, Title VII) provides funding for a variety of programs promoting the use of minority languages in the schools. Civil rights statutes, including The Civil Rights Act of 1964 (Public Law 88-352, Title VI) and The Equal Education Opportunities Act of 1974 (Public Law 93-380) impose an affirmative duty on the schools to give children who speak a minority language an equal educational opportunity by lowering the English-language barriers. The providing of language rights for Deaf students should bring with it appropriate school curricula and materials, teachers who are ethnic models, interpreters, real television access through signed language, and video-telephone communication. But in practice, that effort would require that the public come to understand the Deaf-World as the Deaf-World understands itself. Until this epiphany happens, the Deaf-World can expect scant support from other ethnic groups.

Among the obstacles thwarting a change from the disability construction to the ethnic construction of Deaf people are the numerous professional organizations predicated on the disability construction who wish to own the problem of Deaf children. "To 'own' a social problem is to possess the authority to name that social condition a problem and to suggest what might be done about it" (Gusfield 1989, 433). Consider just two of the many organizations that have Deaf clients. The American Academy of Otolaryngology, with more than 10,000 members, has registered two paid lobbyists in Washington; the American Speech-Language-Hearing Association, with 115,925 members, has three (http://sopr.senate.gov). Members of these organizations collaborate with government officials in approving treatments, in drawing up legislation, and in evaluating proposed research and training activities. The Deaf-World has none of these advantages in seeking to promote an ethnic understanding of being Deaf.

FOUR REASONS TO REJECT THE DISABILITY LABEL

Four reasons justifying why the Deaf-World should reject the disability label make a clear case: it does not reflect the Deaf-World's self-image, it poses greater risk for the Deaf child, it creates a survival risk for the Deaf-World, and it promotes wrong solutions.

The Disability Label "Does Not Compute"

The overwhelming reason to reject the view of culturally Deaf people as members of a disability group concerns how Deaf people see themselves. People who have grown up Deaf and have become integrated into Deaf culture are naturally aware of their biological difference, but they do not, as a rule, see in that difference a reason to consider themselves members of a disability group. This self-perception constitutes a very strong argument for rejecting the disability label because there is no higher authority on how a group should be regarded than the members of the group themselves. Some writers, convinced that the Deaf have a disability and baffled by their refusal to acknowledge it, conclude that Deaf people are simply denying the truth of their disability to avoid stigma (Finkelstein 1981; Gonsoulin 2001; Baynton 2002). But like Deaf people, many people have physical differences that are not accommodated (Zola 1993)—relatively short and tall people, for example—and they, too, deny they have a disability. Surely in doing so they are not simply disingenuously trying to avoid stigma. The gender preferences of gay men and women were at one time viewed as an expression of mental illness. In rejecting that disability categorization, the Gay Rights Movement was not simply trying to avoid a stigma, it was trying instead to promote a new representation of gay men and women that, beyond stigma alone, would be better for them, their families, and the wider society (Conrad and Schneider 1980).

When Gallaudet University's president, I. King Jordan, was asked on a 1990 airing of the television program *Sixty Minutes* whether he would like to be hearing, he replied: "That's almost like asking a black person if he would rather be white. . . . I don't think of myself as missing something or as incomplete. . . . It's a common fallacy if you don't know Deaf people or Deaf issues. You think it's a limitation." Deaf scholars like King Jordan, Tom Humphries, and MJ Bienvenu in the United States and Paddy Ladd in England are not rejecting the disability label because they want to avoid stigma associated with disability (Ladd 2003). That assumption would give them little credit. Rather, they are rejecting it because, as Tom Humphries has said so well, "It doesn't compute" (Humphries 1993, 6, 14). In ASL, the sign whose semantic field most overlaps that of the English *disability* can be glossed in English LIMP-BLIND-ETC. I have asked numerous Deaf informants to give me examples from that category; they have responded by citing people in wheelchairs, blind people, mentally retarded people, and people with cerebral palsy among others, but no informant has ever listed Deaf people, and all reject that group as an example of a disability group when asked.

Further examples of how the disability label does not compute come from Deaf preferences in marriage and childbearing. Like the members of many ethnic groups, culturally Deaf people prefer to socialize with and to marry other members of their cultural group; as noted earlier, the Deaf have one of the highest endogamous marriage rates of any ethnic group (Schein 1989). When it comes to Deaf preferences in childbearing, there are no hard statistics, but in interviews with the press and with me, Deaf parents have expressed a wish for children like themselves—much as all parents do who do not see themselves as disabled. "I want my daughter to be like me, to be Deaf," one expectant Deaf mother declared in an interview with the *Boston Globe*. She explained that she comes from a large Deaf family, all of whom had hoped that her baby would be born Deaf (Saltus 1989; also see Mills 2002). Other expectant Deaf parents reportedly say it would be fine either way, Deaf or hearing. These views contrast sharply with the tendency of disability groups. A study of blind people, for example, reported that they tend to shun the company of other blind people, associate with one another only when there are specific reasons for doing so, seek sighted mates, and do not wish to transmit their blindness to their children (Deshen 1992). Leaders of the disability rights movement call for ambivalence: they want their physical difference valued, as a part of who they are; at the same time, they do not wish to see more children and adults with disabilities in the world (Abberley 1987; Lane 1995).

We should not be surprised that Deaf people want Deaf spouses, welcome Deaf children, and prefer to be together with other culturally Deaf people in clubs, in school, at work if possible, in leisure activities, in political action, in sports, and so on—in short, that they see being Deaf as an inherent good. Ethnic groups characteristically value their physical difference—from the pygmies of the Ituri forest in Central Africa to the tall pale inhabitants of, say, Finland—do they not? Of course they do, so it is perfectly expected that culturally Deaf people positively value the Deaf difference and that hearing folks find in their own cultures a preference for hearing bodies, despite their poorer performance on some visual processing tasks compared with those who are Deaf (Lane 2004a).

Thus, embracing the disability label in hopes that it might assist Deaf people in gaining more of their rights is fundamentally flawed because Deaf people do not believe they are disabled. For Deaf people to surrender to how others define them is to misrepresent themselves. And that is the first reason to reject the disability label.

The Disability Label Poses Greater Risk for the Deaf Child

There are many penalties for misrepresenting the Deaf-World's identity, for allowing the disability label. An important penalty concerns the risk to the Deaf child. It appears that children are at greater medical and surgical risk when their bodies differ from their parents' in important ways that age alone does not explain. Parents want children like themselves, and if those children are significantly unlike them, they will listen to the doctors who say they can reduce or eliminate the difference, sometimes harming the child in the process. It is very tempting to locate the source of the social stigma with the child rather than with the society; after all, the child is right there and is much more manageable than an entire society. Moreover, the technologies of normalization are knocking at the door. However, the medicalization of difference deflects us from the real issue, which is the stigmatizing of difference in our society. When children who have undergone surgical normalizing later become adults, many of them decry what was done to them as children.

For example, it has been the practice in the United States to operate on children with ambiguous genitalia, most often carving a vagina in male children because the surgical methods are not available to create a suitable penis. Once grown to adulthood, these and other intersexuals have been campaigning to dissuade urologists from continuing to perform this maiming surgery on children (Dreger 1998). Little People, when their parents are not dwarfs, are frequently subjected as children to bone-breaking surgery for limb lengthening. It is painful. It is risky. It is incapacitating. At best, it places the child in a no-man's-land, neither short as a dwarf nor average size, and most adult dwarfs are utterly opposed to the surgery (Kennedy 2003). There are many more victims of the medical-surgical imperative. One thinks of the horrors such as frontal lobotomy visited on the mentally ill (Valenstein 1986) and those such as deconditioning visited on homosexuals (Conrad and Schneider 1980). Not all medical intervention in social issues is bad, of course; sometimes, it serves us well and it derives great prestige from doing so, which is why it overreaches at times and why we have to be wary of its abuse. Consider the issues in relation to cochlear implants.

Cochlear Implant Surgery
Today, the Deaf child who is labeled as having a disability is placed at risk for interventions like cochlear implant surgery. Cochlear implant surgery lasts about

three-and-a-half hours under general anesthesia and requires hospitalization from two to four days. A broad crescent-shaped incision is made behind the operated ear, and the skin flap is elevated. A piece of temporalis muscle is removed. A depression is drilled in the skull and is reamed to make a seat for the internal electrical coil of the cochlear implant. A section of the mastoid bone is removed to expose the middle ear cavity. Further drilling exposes the membrane of the round window on the inner ear. Observing the procedure under a microscope, the surgeon pierces the membrane. A wire about 18 mm long is pushed through the opening. The wire seeks its own path as it moves around and up the coiled inner ear. The microstructure of the inner ear is destroyed; if there was any residual hearing in the ear, it, too, is likely destroyed. The auditory nerve itself is unlikely to be damaged, however, and the implant stimulates the auditory nerve directly. The internal coil is then sutured into place. Finally, the skin is sewn back over the coil. The surgery has clear risks and dubious benefits.

Clear risks. The surgery and general anesthesia entail medical and surgical risks. The incidence of bacterial meningitis in implanted children is thirty times higher than in age-matched unimplanted children (Daneshi et al. 2000; Reefhuis et al. 2003). Other risks include anesthesia risk (Svirsky, Teoh, and Neuburger, 2004), loss of vestibular function (Huygen et al. 1995), cerebrospinal fluid leak (Reefhuis et al. 2003), facial nerve stimulation and injury (Kelsall et al. 1997), and damage to the carotid artery (Gastman et al. 2002). The surgery can have fatal consequences (Jalbert 2003). Nine out of ten candidates for pediatric implant surgery, those with no or little usable hearing, were born Deaf (Center for Assessment 1992; Allen, Rawlings, and Remington 1994). Such children rarely receive the main benefit sought: fluency in a spoken language (Lane and Bahan 1998). Compounding the harm, special educators who work with the surgical team commonly urge oral educational programs on the parents and discourage signed language use (Tye-Murray 1992). If implanted children are unable to learn spoken English and are prevented from mastering American Sign Language, then they will remain languageless for many years. Developmental milestones for signed languages are similar to those for spoken languages, and the later the acquisition of ASL, the poorer its mastery on the average (Newport 1990; Mayberry and Eichen 1991; Petitto 1993). It is inexcusable to leave a child without fluent language for years on end. Medicine is coming to realize that it is the overall quality of life of the person, and not just the concerned organ, that must be considered (Reisenberg and Glass 1989).

Dubious benefits. Advocates for childhood implantation acknowledge that "implants do not restore normal hearing" and that, after the operation, "long-term habilitation continues to be essential" (Balkany et al. 2002, 356). According to a recent report, 59 percent of implanted children are judged by their parents to be behind their hearing peers in reading and 37 percent, behind in math (Christiansen and Leigh 2004). It seems unlikely these children will be full-fledged members of the hearing world (Lane and Bahan 1998; Lane 1999).

We know that early acquisition of American Sign Language facilitates later mastery of English (Padden and Ramsey 2000; Strong and Prinz 1997). This linguistic intervention might deliver greater English mastery than implant surgery; the comparison study has not been done. On the contrary, every study that has compared the performance of children who have cochlear implants with an unimplanted control group used controls that apparently had not mastered any language (see, for example, the literature review in Geers, Nicholas, and Sedey 2003).

Ethics of Childhood Implant Surgery

Thus, the surgery remains innovative despite more than a decade of use because research on language benefit and its parameters is very much a work in progress (see, for example, Svirsky, Teoh, and Neuburger 2004). Then, too, there is no body of knowledge on the effects of the implant on educational achievement, social identity, or psychological adjustment. Optional innovative surgery on children is ethically problematic (Lane and Grodin 1997).

It is hard to see how the pediatric implant surgeon can obtain informed consent from the parent, who is acting as moral agent for his or her child. Among the requirements for informed consent are a description of risks, but the physician cannot explain the risks of disturbed psychological, social, and linguistic development because these have not been assessed by scientific research. Further, the surgeon must describe the benefits to be reasonably expected from pediatric cochlear implant surgery, but the variability of outcomes is so great that it is difficult to say what benefit any individual child will obtain. Of course, if the risks of cochlear implant surgery and its associated speech therapy and oral education outweigh the benefits, then it should not be performed.

True informed consent would require the surgeon to disclose alternative procedures that might be advantageous for the subject, for example, early association with Deaf peers and adults to ensure timely language acquisition, but otologists and audiologists are often uninformed about the Deaf-World and its language and are disinclined to see that as an alternative.

Parents, too, face obstacles to informed consent. Recognition that parents indeed face these obstacles is not to challenge the parents' legal and moral right to make decisions for their children, as some writers have disingenuously claimed (Hyde, 1994; Balkany, Hodges, and Goodman 1999; Eisenman 1999). For surgeons, parental choice is a touchstone because they share with most parents a medical model of the Deaf child's status; thus, parental choice is surgeon's choice. Would the surgeons be as eager to extol parental choice if most parents declined the surgery?

The ethical basis for the parent acting as surrogate for the child is predicated on the assumption that the surrogate knows the child or is close to his or her cultural or ethical values. The surrogate's choices should approximate what the patient would have wanted were he or she able to express a choice (Ramsey 1970). Unfortunately, hearing parents often do not know the patient because they have lacked a common language with their Deaf child. In fact, most Deaf children would likely refuse that consent to surgery if they were old enough to decide. We infer that conclusion because Deaf adults, who were once Deaf children but are now old enough to make a considered decision, are overwhelmingly opposed to pediatric implant surgery. Numerous Deaf organizations worldwide and the World Federation of the Deaf have formally protested childhood implant surgery (Lane 1994). The National Association of the Deaf in the United States takes the position that Deaf children are healthy babies; of course, surgery should not be performed on a healthy child. Their statement says in part,

Many within the medical profession continue to view deafness essentially as a disability and an abnormality and believe that deaf and hard of hearing individuals need to be 'fixed' by cochlear implants. This pathological view must be challenged and corrected by greater exposure to and interaction with well-adjusted and successful deaf and hard of hearing individuals. (National Association of the Deaf 2000)

If medical and surgical procedures used with children who are Deaf—or inter-sexuals or dwarfs—required informed consent from adults who were like the child, then they would almost never take place! And when the parents are like the child, in fact, they rarely take place.

Hearing parents of a Deaf child confront a challenge that is in some ways not unlike that faced by parents who adopt transracially. Both sets of parents have physical attributes markedly different from their children, and in both cases, the children would normally become members of ethnic groups different from their parents. Are white foster parents of a black child, then, obliged to consider, or well-advised to consider, the views and interests of the black community? Many social workers believe so (Chimezie 1975).

Likewise, hearing parents of a Deaf child would have much to gain from consulting Deaf adults. Deaf parents commonly raise Deaf and hearing children perfectly well without any surgery or other intervention by professionals. In fact, abundant research evidence indicates that they do a better job on the average than hearing parents of Deaf children do, and hearing parents often have professional intervention (Lane, Hoffmeister, and Bahan 1996; Lane 1999). So it is clear that it would be a needless error to place Deaf children at risk of the medical-surgical imperative by labeling the Deaf as a disability group. (Granted there are disability groups who protest excessive surgical and medical intervention, but that is not a reasonable basis for considering Deaf children disabled.)

Why would such heroic medicine be practiced on young Deaf children who, moreover, cannot give their consent? The plight of Deaf children must be seen as truly desperate to warrant such action. In hearing society, deafness is indeed stigmatized. Sociologist Erving Goffman has distinguished three kinds of stigma: physical, characterological, and tribal. "There is only one complete, unblushing male in America," he explained. "[He is] a young, married, white urban northern heterosexual Protestant father of college education, fully employed, of good complexion, weight, and height, and a recent record in sports" (Goffman 1963, 128). Any deviation is likely to entail a stigma, and society tends to impute many when it finds a single one.

The layperson is misled not only by the common stigma associated with Deaf people in hearing society but also, as countless parents of Deaf children have been misled, by some practitioners in fields such as otology, audiology and special education, and rehabilitation—the technologies of normalization, who paint the consequences of being Deaf in the most negative terms possible, thereby reaffirming the need for their services. Witness this outlandish claim by a pediatric implant team: "Deafness is the most disabling of disabilities" (Balkany, Hodges, and Goodman 1996, 751). Cochlear implants are relatively new, but they are the latest stage in a long history in which the technologies of normalization have undertaken to make Deaf people more like hearing people. Each Deaf child in America is the scion of Deaf people across the ages; he or she receives a Deaf heritage and passes it on. Each Deaf child, then, experiences twice over the attempts by hearing people to change Deaf people, first as a theme of Deaf history and second as a theme of personal history. Consequently, rare is the Deaf child today in America who has not been subjected to such normalizing attempts—through surgery, through medicine, through therapy, through sacrificing education for sham speech—and all these efforts, nearly always a failure for the nine out of ten Deaf children born Deaf.

When the first school for the Deaf in the Western world was established in Paris during the Enlightenment, painful surgical experiments on its pupils helped its resident doctor gain the title of founder of otology. His successor captured the view of Deaf children held by many surgeons then, as now; he wrote: "The Deaf believe that they are our equals in all respects. We should be generous and not destroy that illusion. But whatever they believe, deafness is an infirmity and we should repair it whether the person who has it is disturbed by it or not" (Menière 1853 quoted in Houdin 1855, 14). Like the members of other ethnic minorities, Deaf people are generally not disturbed by their identity, despite the need to struggle for their rights. Culturally Deaf people have always thought, and think today, that being Deaf is a perfectly good way to be, as good as hearing, perhaps better.

The Disability Label Creates a Survival Risk for the Deaf-World

A third argument against the disability label for the Deaf-World concerns the risk to the Deaf-World as a whole if that representation prevails. A majority of people in the Deaf-World have inherited their ethnicity, as stated earlier. Deaf inheritance and a failure to understand the ethnic status of culturally Deaf people has historically, and at present, placed the Deaf-World in jeopardy of ethnocide and even genocide. Despite surgical and medical experiments on large numbers of Deaf children in the nineteenth century, medicine made no inroads against the Deaf-World as a whole. However, developments in biology in the late nineteenth century gave rise to the eugenics movement, which sought through selective breeding to improve the race and eliminate not only the Deaf-World but also other groups considered undesirable. From the point of view of the variety of humankind favored by selective breeding, the practice is eugenic; from the point of view of the varieties disfavored, it is genocidal.

The most famous advocate of regulating Deaf marriage to reduce Deaf childbirth was one of the founders of oral education in America, Alexander Graham Bell, who devoted his great wealth and prestige to these eugenic measures (Lane 1984). When the American Breeders Association created a section on eugenics "to emphasize the value of superior blood and the menace to society of inferior blood," Bell agreed to serve. He engaged the issue of eugenics and the Deaf population beginning in the 1880s. Signed language and residential schools were creating a Deaf community, he warned, in which Deaf people intermarried and reproduced, a situation fraught with danger to the rest of society. He sounded the alarm in his *Memoir upon the Formation of a Deaf Variety of the Human Race*, presented to the National Academy of Sciences in 1883. Because there are familial patterns of deafness, Bell wrote, "It is to be feared that the intermarriage of such persons would be attended by calamitous results to their off-spring" (Bell 1883, 11). Bell argued, with breathtaking hubris, that to avoid this calamity, we must "commence our efforts on behalf of the deaf-mute by changing his social environment" (46). Residential schools, where most Deaf children acquired language, identity, and a life partner, should be closed and Deaf people educated in small day schools, he recommended. Signed language should be banished; Deaf teachers, fired. Bell's *Memoir* received wide newspaper coverage. Bell's actions led many to believe that there would be, or already were, laws prohibiting Deaf marriage. There was much consternation among Deaf people contemplating marriage. Some hearing parents of Deaf children chose to have their children sterilized (Mitchell 1971).

A 1912 report from Bell's eugenics section of the Breeders' Association cites his census of blind and Deaf persons and lists "socially unfit" classes to "be eliminated from the human stock" (American Genetic Association 1912, 3). The model eugenic law (1912, 3) called for the sterilization of feebleminded, insane, criminalistic ("including the delinquent and the wayward"), epileptic, inebriate, diseased, blind, Deaf, deformed and dependent people ("including orphans, ne'er-do-wells, the homeless, tramps and paupers"). By the time of World War I, sixteen states in the United States had sterilization laws in force; by 1940, thirty states had such laws (Haller 1963). Physicians were actively involved in this eugenics movement (May and Hughes 1987).

The eugenics movement as it concerned Deaf people worldwide has only recently been receiving the study it deserves (Biesold 1999; Schuchman and Ryan 2002). When National Socialism came to power in Germany, teachers of Deaf students advocated adherence to the hereditary purity laws, including the sterilization of congenitally Deaf people. Deaf school children were required to prepare family trees, and the school reported those children who were congenitally Deaf or who had a Deaf relative to the department of health for possible sterilization (Muhs 1996).

The German sterilization law that went into effect in 1934 provided that "Those hereditarily sick may be made unfruitful (sterilized) through surgical intervention. . . . The hereditary sick, in the sense of this law, is a person who suffers from one of the following diseases . . . hereditary deafness" (Peter 1934, 187). The 1933 German census showed forty-five thousand "deaf and dumb" persons in a total population of more than 66 million. An estimated seventeen thousand of these Deaf Germans, a third of them minors, were sterilized. In nine percent of the cases, sterilization was accompanied by forced abortion. An additional sixteen hundred Deaf people were exterminated in concentration camps in the 1940s; they were considered "useless eaters," whose lives were unworthy of being lived (Higgins 1993; Biesold 1999). As in the United States, the medical profession was the certifying authority for forced sterilization.

Deaf Eugenics Today
Audiometric testing, labeling, special-needs schooling, genetic research and counseling, surgery and reproductive control all are means of currently or potentially exercising power over the Deaf body. In 1992, researchers at Boston University announced that they had identified the so-called "genetic error" responsible for

a common type of inherited deafness, Waardenburg's Syndrome. The director of the National Institute on Deafness and Other Communication Disorders (note the label *Other Communication Disorders*) called the finding a "major breakthrough that will improve diagnosis and genetic counseling and ultimately lead to substitution therapy or gene transfer therapy" (*Deaf Community News* 992, 6; *The New York Times* 1992, 141). The goal of such efforts as gene transfer therapy is, of course, to reduce Deaf births, ultimately altogether. Thus, a new form of medical eugenics applied to Deaf people is envisioned, in this case, by an agency of the U.S. government. The primary characteristics to be eliminated among Deaf people with this particular genetic background are numerous Deaf relatives, signed language fluency, facial features such as widely spaced eyebrows, and coloring features such as white forelock and freckling (Fraser 1976).

Imagine the uproar if medical scientists trumpeted a similar breakthrough for any other ethnic minority, promising a reduction in that ethnic group's children—for example, promising fewer Navajos, fewer Jews, whatever the ethnic group. The Australian government indeed undertook a decades-long eugenic program to eliminate its aboriginal peoples by placing their children in white-owned boarding houses in the city where it was hoped the children eventually would marry white people and have white children. In 1997, a government commission of inquiry classified these and other measures as genocide (National Inquiry 1997). Under international law, an activity that has the foreseeable effect of diminishing or eradicating a minority group, even if it is undertaken for other reasons and is not highly effective, is guilty of genocide (United Nations 1948; National Inquiry 1997). Why do governments fail to apply this moral principle and law to the Deaf? Americans fail to see the danger of pursuing a genocidal program in this instance because most Americans see Deaf people as having a disability arising from an impairment. And the goal of eradicating a disability, although it may be in some circumstances unwise and unethical, is not seen as genocide.

If culturally Deaf people were understood to be an ethnic group, they would have the protections offered to such groups. It is widely held as an ethical principle that the preservation of minority cultures is a good. The variety of humankind and cultures enriches all cultures and contributes to the biological, social, and psychological well-being of humankind. Laws and covenants such as the United Nations' *Declaration on the Rights of Persons Belonging to National or Ethnic, Religious and Linguistic Minorities* (United Nations 1992), are founded on a belief in the value of protecting minority cultures. The Declaration calls on states to foster their linguistic minorities and ensure that children and adults have adequate opportunities to learn the minority language. It further affirms the right of such minorities to enjoy their culture and language and to participate in decisions on the national level that affect them. Programs that substantially diminish minority cultures are engaged in ethnocide and may constitute crimes against humanity.

Cochlear Implants and Controlling the Deaf Body

Among the biological means sought for regulating and, ultimately, eliminating Deaf culture, language, and people, cochlear implants have historical antecedents in medical experimentation on Deaf children and in reproductive regulation of Deaf adults. We have seen abundant scientific evidence for classifying the Deaf-World as an ethnic group. Many Americans, perhaps most, would agree that society should not seek the scientific tools nor use them, if available, to change a child biologically so he or she will belong to the majority rather than the minority—even if society believes that this biological engineering might reduce the burdens the child will bear as a member of a minority. Even if children destined to be members of the African-American or Hispanic-American or Native-American or Deaf-American cultures could be somehow biologically converted into white, Caucasian, hearing males, even if society could accomplish this act, it should not. Here lies the answer to bioethicist Dena Davis, who has argued that it would be wrong to withhold a perfect implant from a Deaf child because the Deaf-World is a limiting one and withholding her implant would reduce the child's possibilities in life; it would violate her right to an "open future" (Davis 1997, 256). It is true that minority members frequently have a less open future than majority members, yet we all would agree that surgery that is sought merely to help a child "pass" as a member of the majority or simply to facilitate learning the majority language is unethical. Why does Dr. Davis endorse such surgery on the Deaf child but not on the black one? Because she continues to see the Deaf child as disabled.

Surgeons have made the claim that a Deaf child is not yet a member of the Deaf-World and, thus, a program of implanting Deaf children should not be viewed as undermining that ethnic minority (Cohen 1994). In fact, these surgeons imply that Deaf people should mind their own business because young Deaf children of hearing parents are not culturally Deaf. Because much turns on this point, it is worth considering the logic of how we make cultural assignments. Three possible premises seem possible: the infant belongs to no culture at all until a certain age or stage of development; the infant has the culture of his or her parents from birth; or the infant has the cultural affiliation he or she will normally acquire. Now it is a fact that the child is launched at the moment of birth onto a trajectory that, depending on the child's makeup and environment, will normally lead him or her to master a particular language and culture natively. It is this potentiality in the newborn Native-American child, for example, that leads us to say that child *is* Native American (not *will be*)—even though the child has not yet acquired the language and culture that go with that cultural attribution. In making this attribution, we would not ask first about the parents' culture. Their physical makeup and culture (their ethnicity), though usually consonant with their child's, does not itself decide the child's cultural assignment; it is the makeup of the child that does. With adoptive parents or even a surrogate mother, the child with Native-American constitution would be called Native American. Thus, a program of adopting such infants into Caucasian homes would be guilty of undermining Native-American culture, and its proponents could not deny it on the grounds that the children had not yet learned that culture and its language.

Ethicist Dena Davis, responding to my article with Michael Grodin titled "Ethical Issues in Cochlear Implant Surgery" (Lane and Grodin 1997), disputes these claims: "I reject the notion that physical characteristics . . . constitute cultural membership" (Davis 1997, 254). However, it is undeniable that culture and physical characteristics are at times obviously intertwined and mutually reliant. Consider the adaptation of culture to physical characteristics by returning to the example of the forest dwellers. Their culture is very much associated with their height in its coupling to their environment. Because pygmies are short, they have low caloric requirements and can move more rapidly through the dense forest.

Their small body mass and speed apparently underpin their method of food gathering and their method of food gathering underpins their cooperative culture. Pygmies hunt in groups of six or seven families, each with its own hunting net; the women and children drive the animals into the long circle of nets joined end to end, and the take is shared. In view of net hunting, close reciprocal collaboration is needed in many facets of life. That may be the reason that pygmy families in a hunting group live together in a closed circle of small conical huts. The maintenance of law is also a cooperative affair, as is worship. All these pygmy cultural issues—cooperative hunting, living, justice, and worship—seem to have their roots in the pygmies' physical characteristics.

Consider, too, a more widespread example of physical characteristics associated with culture—gender, which has profound consequences for acculturation in most of the nations of the world, if not all. It is this association between physical characteristics and culture that no doubt leads to the principle of cultural attribution stated above: infants have the culture their makeup would normally yield. An intervention such as transracial adoption can override the expected outcome (Nunes 2001). In that case, the black child, for example, might not have the opportunity to acquire the language and culture of his ethnic group, but he or she remains black nonetheless, according to our society's rules of cultural attribution. The same phenomenon occurs with Deaf children; they commonly have delayed access to Deaf culture and language because their parents are unable or disinclined to give them that access. Only a minority of black children find themselves in this predicament; a majority of Deaf children do.

Hence the newborn Deaf child *is* culturally Deaf (hence my use of capital-D *Deaf*) and a program of implanting Deaf children does indeed undermine that ethnic minority. Suppose there were perfect implants and these were given to Deaf children routinely. If there were no Deaf children, then there would be no Deaf-World. The Deaf infant may not yet have acquired the language and culture that are, given its makeup, its natural right and heritage, those it will prize as an adult (because most born Deaf people do), but the child's life trajectory is surely headed there because he or she uses vision almost exclusively and communicates visually, not aurally. The child may have hearing biological parents, but this child is not a hearing person either in principle, as we have seen, or in practice. As a matter of practice, if the parents cannot communicate fluently with their child, they will be severely hampered in teaching the child their language and culture, and the child can never acquire them natively, without instruction, as a hearing child would. However adept hearing parents may be, they cannot model Deaf adulthood, only hearing adulthood, and a child who relies primarily on vision will never develop into a hearing person, not even remotely. Conversely, the parents will never be culturally Deaf. Thus, uncommon as it may be among other cultures, Deaf children and their parents very often do not share the same cultural membership.

The U.S. Indian Child Welfare Act of 1978 (25 U.S.C. §§ 1901-63) was passed at a time when the survival of Native-American cultures was considered threatened by very high rates of transracial adoption. The act was designed to prevent the undermining of Native American tribes, stating that "it is the policy of this nation to protect the best interests of Indian children and to promote the stability and security of Indian tribes" (Simon and Altstein 1992, 18–19). The social issues leading to the act were in many ways specific to that minority, but the dual principle the Congress recognized was general: protect the child *and* protect the ethnic group. The Supreme Court ruled that lower courts must consider not only the best interests of the child but also the best interests of the particular Indian tribe (Simon and Altstein 1992). Do the ethical principles applied here not apply equally well to other ethnic groups, including the Deaf-World?

As members of a stigmatized minority, Deaf children's lives will be full of challenge, but by the same token, they have a special contribution to make to their own community and the larger society. The more children who are born Deaf are viewed, not as members of a minority culture, but as disabled, then the more society is prepared to conduct surgery of unproven benefit and unassessed risk, ignoring the harm that is done to the child's ethnic group. The representation of Deaf people determines the outcome of society's ethical judgment.

The Disability Label Promotes Wrong Solutions

Because they are an ethnic group whose language and mores were long disparaged, Deaf people commonly feel solidarity with other oppressed groups, the more so as the Deaf-World includes groups such as people with disabilities, seniors, women, blacks, and so on. Deaf people have special reasons for solidarity with hard of hearing and late-deafened people; their combined numbers have created services, commissions, and laws that the Deaf-World alone probably could not have achieved. Solidarity, yes, but when culturally Deaf people allow their ethnic identity to be subsumed under the construct of disability, they set themselves up for wrong solutions and bitter disappointments. After all, members of the Deaf-World differ from disabled people in their language and cultural experience, in their body of knowledge, in their system of rules and values, and in their models for selfhood.

If the Deaf-World were to embrace a disability identity, it would encourage an understanding from which grow solutions that Deaf people oppose. Priorities of the disabilities rights movement include better medical care, rehabilitation services, and personal assistance services (Shapiro 1993). Deaf people do not attach particular importance to any of these services and, instead, campaign for acceptance of their language as well as better and more interpreters. The disability rights movement seeks independence for people with disabilities whereas Deaf people cherish interdependence with other Deaf people. These differences in values and priorities far outweigh the areas such as fighting job discrimination in which Deaf goals are potentially advanced by joining ranks with disability groups.

Disability advocates think of Deaf children as disabled and, thus, those advocates have endeavored to close the special schools, where Deaf children gained language and a proud identity, and to absurdly plunge Deaf children into hearing classrooms and a thoroughly exclusionary environment called "inclusion" (Lane 2004b). Precisely because government is allowed to proceed with a disability construction of Deaf ethnicity, the U.S. Office of Bilingual Education and Minority Language Affairs does not provide special resources for schools with large numbers of children whose best language is ASL, even though the law requires it to do so for schools with large numbers of students whose best language is not English.

As explained earlier, there are landmark court rulings in the United States under the Civil Rights Act and the Equal Educational Opportunities Act that require schools with children who have "limited English proficiency" to provide instruction initially using the children's native language. The *Code of Federal Regulations* quite sensibly defines "native language" as the language normally used by the individual (*Code of Federal Regulations*, Title 34, Subtitle B, Chapter V, Part 500.4, 7-1-87 ed.). Deaf children's native language is signed language (provided, of course, that they are given an opportunity to acquire it). Deaf children have a particularly strong claim on bilingual education because, like many members of other ethnic groups but more so, they will never make a transition to full use of English and will always require an important part of their instruction in their best language. Again, because of the disability construction of Deaf people, those laws have not been applied to children who use ASL. Further, because of the disability construction, the teachers most able to communicate with America's Deaf children are excluded from the profession on the grounds that they have a disqualifying disability. And because lawmakers see Deaf people as disabled, Congress passed a law, prompted by the Deaf revolution at Gallaudet University, not recognizing ASL as a language of instruction or the Deaf-World as an ethnic minority but, instead, establishing another institute of *health* —The National Institute on Deafness and Other Communication Disorders, operated by the troubled-persons industry, and sponsoring research to reduce the numbers of Deaf people.

This paper has presented a case that the signed-language-using minority in the United States, the Deaf-World, is best viewed as an ethnic group, and it has cited reasons why it is inappropriate to view the Deaf-World as a disability group: Deaf people themselves do not believe they have a disability; the disability construction brings with it needless medical and surgical risks for the Deaf child; it also endangers the future of the Deaf-World; and finally, the disability construction brings bad solutions to real problems because it is predicated on a misunderstanding.

All of these objections to the disability construction of culturally Deaf people also apply to the proposal that Deaf people be understood as both an ethnic group and a disability group at the same time. Taking up such a position would weaken the Deaf-World claim on ethnicity (is there any other ethnic group that is a disability group?) while inviting the risks and wrong solutions described above. The ethically troubling practices in which surgeons, scientists, and educators are engaged—operating on healthy Deaf children, seeking the means to diminish and ultimately eradicate the Deaf-World, opposing the Deaf child's right to full and fluent language—exist because this ethnic group is misunderstood as a disability group. These practices will not be avoided by affirming, contrary to the group's own judgment, that it is a disability group but also an ethnic group.

How we ultimately resolve these ethical issues goes well beyond Deaf people; our response will say a great deal about what kind of society we are and the kind of society in which we wish to live. Difference and diversity not only have evolutionary significance but also, I would argue, are a major part of what gives life its richness and meaning; ethnic diversity is a basic human good, and to choose to be with one's own kind is a fundamental right. There is reason for hope: society *can* adopt a different understanding of a people. Native Americans were once seen as savages; black Americans, as property; women, as utterly dependent. The case for Deaf ethnicity that has been built by the social sciences is powerful. Increasingly, linguists take account of ASL; sociologists, of the social structure of the Deaf-World; historians, of its history; educators, of its culture and so on. Still, the task remains to reform those other professions that have an outdated understanding or a representation that suits their agenda but not that of Deaf people. The challenge to the professions that seek to be of service to Deaf children and adults is to replace the normativeness of medicine with the curiosity of ethnography.

REFERENCES

Abberley, P. 1987. The Concept of oppression and the development of a social theory of disability. *Disability, Handicap and Society*, 2: 5–19.

Allen, T. E., B. W. Rawlings, and E. Remington. 1994. Demographic and audiologic profiles of deaf children in Texas with cochlear implants. *American Annals of the Deaf*, 138: 260–66.

American Genetic Association, Eugenics Section. 1912. American sterilization laws. Preliminary report of the committee of the eugenics section of the American Breeders Association to study and to report on the best practical means for cutting off the defective germ plasm in the human population. London: Eugenics Educational Society.

Bahan, B. 2005. Memoir upon the formation of a visual variety of the human race. In *Deaf studies today*, ed. B. K. Eldredge, D. Stringham, and M. Wilding-Diaz, 17–35. Orem, Utah: Utah Valley State College.

Balkany, T. J., A. V. Hodges, A. A. Eshraghi, S. Butts, K. Bricker, J. Lingvai, M. Polak, and J. King. 2002. Cochlear implants in children: A review. *Acta Otolaryngologica* (Stockholm) 122: 356–62.

Balkany, T., A. Hodges, and K. Goodman. 1996. Ethics of cochlear implantation in young children. *Otolaryngology—Head and Neck Surgery* 114: 748–55.

———. 1999. Authors' reply [to Lane and Bahan]. *Otolaryngology—Head and Neck Surgery* 121: 673–75.

Barth, F. 1969. *Ethnic groups and boundaries.* Boston: Little Brown.

Baynton, D. 2000. Bodies and environments. In *Employment, disability and the Americans with Disabilities Act*, ed. P. Blanet, 387–411. Evanston, Ill.: Northwestern University Press.

———. 2002. Deafness and disability. Paper presented at the Deaf Studies Think Tank, July 5–7, Gallaudet University, Washington, D.C.

Bell, A. G. 1883. *Memoir upon the formation of a deaf variety of the human race.* Washington, D.C.: Volta Bureau.

Biesold, H. 1999. *Crying hands: Eugenics and deaf people in Nazi Germany.* Trans. W. Sayers. Washington, D.C.: Gallaudet University Press. Translated from the original *Klagende Hande: Betroffenheit und Spatfolgen in Bezug auf das Gesetz zur Verhutung erbkranken Nachwuches, dargestellt am Beispiel der "Taubstummen."* Solms-Oberbiel: Jarick Oberbiel, 1998.

Binnie C. 1994. The future of audiologic rehabilitation: Overview and forecast. In *Research in audiological rehabilitation*, ed. J. P. Gagné and N. Tye-Murray, 13–24. Cedar Falls, Iowa: American Academy of Rehabilitative Audiology.

Bullard, D. 1986. *Islay.* Silver Spring, Md.: TJ Publishers.

Center for Assessment and Demographic Studies, Gallaudet University. 1992. Annual survey of hearing-impaired children and youth 1991–1992: Age at onset of deafness for students with profound hearing losses. Washington, D.C.: Gallaudet University.

Chimezie, A. 1975. Transracial adoption of black children. *Social Work* 20: 296–301.

Christiansen, J. B., and I. W. Leigh. 2004. Children with cochlear implants: Changing parent and Deaf community perspectives. *Archives of Otolaryngology— Head and Neck Surgery* 130: 673–77.

Cohen, N. 1994. The ethics of cochlear implants in young children. *American Journal of Otology* 15: 2.

Conrad, P., and J. Schneider. 1980. *Deviance and medicalization.* Columbus Ohio: Merrill.

Daneshi, A., M. Farhadi, H. Emamjomeh, and S. Hasanzadeh. 2000. Management and the control of gusher during cochlear implant surgery. *Advances in Otorhino-Laryngology* 57: 120–22.

Davis, D. S. 1997. Cochlear implants and the claims of culture? A response to Lane and Grodin. *Kennedy Institute of Ethics Journal* 7: 253–58.

Davis, L. 2002. Postdeafness. Paper presented at the Deaf Studies Think Tank, July 5–7, Gallaudet University, Washington, D.C.

Deaf Community News. 1992. Boston University team finds genetic cause of Waardenburg Syndrome. March.

Deshen, S. 1992. *Blind people.* Albany, N.Y.: State University of New York Press.

Downie, A. B., J. Mulligan, E. S. McCaughey, R. J. Stratford, P. R. Betts, and L. D. Voss. 1996. Psychological response to treatment in short normal children. *Archives of Disorders of Childhood* 76: 92–95.

Dreger, A. 1998. *Hermaphrodites and the medical invention of sex.* Cambridge: Harvard University Press.

Eisenman, D. J. 1999. To the editor [a reply to Lane and Bahan]. *Otolaryngology— Head and Neck Surgery* 121: 670–71.

Erting, C. 1978. Language policy and Deaf ethnicity in the United States. *Sign Language Studies* 19: 139–52.

———. 1982. Deafness, communication and social identity: An anthropological analysis of interaction among parents, teachers and deaf children in a preschool. Ph.D. diss., Anthropology Department, American University, Washington, D.C.

Finkelstein, V. 1981. Disability and the helper-helped relationship. In *Handicap in a social world,* ed. A. Brechin, P. Liddiard, and J. Swain, 58–64. Sevenoaks, Kent: Hodder and Stoughton in association with Open University Press.

———. 1991 "We" are not disabled, "you" are. In *Constructing Deafness,* ed. S. Gregory and G. M. Hartley, 265–71. London: Pinter.

Fishman, J. 1977. Language and ethnicity. In *Language, ethnicity, and intergroup relations,* ed. H. Giles, 15–57. New York, N.Y.: Academic Press.

———. 1982. A critique of six papers on the socialization of the deaf child. In *Conference highlights: National research conference on the social aspects of deafness,* ed. J. B. Christiansen, 6–20. Washington, D.C.: Gallaudet College.

———. 1989. *Language and ethnicity in minority sociolinguistic perspective.* Philadelphia, Penn.: Multilingual Matters.

Foucault, M. 1980. *Power/Knowledge: Selected interviews and other writings, 1972–1977.* Brighton, Sussex: Harvester Press.

Fraser, G. R. 1976. *The causes of profound deafness in childhood.* Baltimore: Johns Hopkins Press.

Gastman, B. R., B. E. Hirsch, I. Sando, M. B. Fukui, and M. L. Wargo. 2002. The potential risk of carotid injury in cochlear implant surgery. *Laryngoscope* 112: 262–66.

Geers, A. E., J. G. Nicholas, and A. L. Sedey. 2003. Language skills of children with early cochlear implantation. *Ear and Hearing* 24 (Suppl.): 46S–58S.

Gelb, S. A. 1987. Social deviance and the "discovery" of the moron. *Disability, Handicap and Society* 2: 247–58.

Goffman, E. 1963. *Stigma: Notes on the management of spoiled identity.* Englewood Cliffs, N.J.: Prentice-Hall.

Gonsoulin, T. P. 2001. Cochlear implant/Deaf-World dispute: Different bottom elephants. *Otolaryngology—Head and Neck Surgery* 125: 552–56.

Gusfield, J. 1982. Deviance in the welfare state: The alcoholism profession and the entitlements of stigma. In *Research in social problems and public policy*, Vol. 2, ed. M. Lewis, 1–20. Greenwich Conn.: JAI Press.

———. 1984. On the side: Practical action and social constructivism in social problems theory. In *Studies in the sociology of social problems*, ed. J. Schneider and J. Kitsuse, 31–51. Rutgers: Ablex.

———. 1989. Constructing the ownership of social problems: Fun and profit in the welfare state. *Social Problems* 36: 431–41.

Haller, M. 1963. *Eugenics: Hereditarian attitudes in American thought.* New Brunswick, N.J.: Rutgers University Press.

Higgins, W., ed. 1993. La parole des sourds. *Psychoanalystes* 46–47: 1–216.

Humphries T. 1993. Deaf culture and cultures. In *Multicultural issues in deafness*, ed. K. M. Christensen and G. L. Delgado, 3–15. White Plains, N.Y.: Longman.

Huygen, P. L., J. B. Hinderink, P. van den Broek, S. van den Borne, J. P. Brokx, L. H. Mens, and R. J. Admiraal. 1995. The risk of vestibular function loss after intracochlear implantation. *Acta Otolaryngologica* Suppl. 520, part 2: 270–2.

Hyde, M. 1994. Some ethical dimensions of cochlear implantation of deaf children. *Annals of Otology, Rhinology and Laryngology* 166: 19–20.

Jalbert, Y. 2003. Décès suite à un implant cochléaire : Pas un type B. *Canadian Medical Association Journal* 168: 256.

Johnson, R. E., and C. Erting. 1979. Sign, solidarity, and socialization. Paper presented at the meeting of the American Anthropological Association, November, Cincinnati, Ohio.

———. 1982. Linguistic socialization in the context of emergent deaf ethnicity. In *Working papers no. 1: Deaf children and the socialization process*, ed. C. Erting and R. Meisegeier. Washington, D.C.: Sociology Department, Gallaudet College.

———. 1984. Linguistic socialization in the context of emergent Deaf ethnicity. In *Wenner-Gren Foundation working papers in anthropology*, ed. K. Kernan. New York, N.Y.: Wenner-Gren.

———. 1989. Ethnicity and socialization in a classroom for Deaf children. In *The sociolinguistics of the Deaf community*, ed. C. Lucas, 41–84. New York, N.Y.: Academic Press.

Kelsall, D. C., J. K. Shallop, T. G. Brammeier, and E. C. Prenger. 1997. Facial nerve stimulation after Nucleus 22-channel cochlear implantation. *American Journal of Otology* 18: 336–41.

Kennedy, D. 2003. *Little people*. New York, N.Y.: St. Martin's Press.

Ladd, P. 2003. *Understanding deaf culture: In search of deafhood*. London: Multilingual Matters.

Lane, H. 1984. *When the mind hears: A history of the Deaf*. New York: Random House.

———. 1994. The cochlear implant controversy. *World Federation of the Deaf News* (2–3): 22–28.

———. 1995. Constructions of deafness. *Disability and Society* 10: 171–89.

———. 1999. *Mask of benevolence*. 2d ed. San Diego: DawnSignPress.

———. 2004a. *A Deaf artist in early America: The worlds of John Brewster Jr.* Boston: Beacon Press.

———. 2004b. The education of Deaf children: Drowning in the mainstream and the sidestream. In *The illusion of full inclusion: A comprehensive critique of a current special education bandwagon*, ed. J. Kauffman and D. Hallahan, 275–87. Austin, Tex.: Pro-Ed.

Lane, H., and B. Bahan. 1998. Effects of cochlear implantation in young children: A review and a reply from a DEAF-WORLD perspective. *Otolaryngology—Head and Neck Surgery* 119: 297–308.

Lane, H., and M. Grodin. 1997. Ethical Issues in cochlear implant surgery: An exploration into disease, disability, and the best interests of the child. *Kennedy Institute of Ethics Journal* 7: 231–51.

Lane, H., R. Hoffmeister, and B. Bahan. 1996. *A journey into the Deaf-World*. San Diego: DawnSignPress.

Lane, H., R. Pillard, and M. French. 2000. Origins of the American Deaf-World: Assimilating and differentiating societies and their relation to genetic patterning. *Sign Language Studies* 1 (new series): 17–44.

Levesque, J. 1994. It's a Deaf Deaf Deaf-World. *DCARA News* 15: 2.

Markowicz, H., and J. Woodward. 1978. Language and the maintenance of ethnic boundaries in the Deaf community. *Communication and Cognition* 11: 29–37.

May, D., and D. Hughes. 1987. Organizing services for people with mental handicap: The Californian experience. *Disability, Handicap and Society* 2: 213–230.

Mayberry, R., and E. Eichen, E. 1991. The long-lasting advantage of learning sign language in childhood: Another look at the critical period for language acquisition. *Journal of Memory and Language* 30: 486–512.

Menière, P. 1853. *De la guérison de la surdi-mutité et de l'"éducation des sourds-muets. Exposé de la discussion qui a eu lieu a l'Académie Impériale de Médecine, avec notes critiques*. Paris: Bailliere. Cited in Houdin, A. De la surdi-mutité; examen critique et raisonné de la discussion soulevée a l'Académie Impériale de Médecine de Paris, séances des 19 et 26 avril . . . 1853 sur cinq questions. Paris: Lube,1855.

Mills, M. 2002. An interview with Sharon Ridgway. *The Guardian*, April 9.

Mindess, A. 1999. *Reading between the signs: Intercultural communication for sign language interpreters*. Yarmouth, Maine: Intercultural Press.

Mitchell, S. H. 1971. The haunting influence of Alexander Graham Bell. *American Annals of the Deaf* 116: 349–56.

Muhs, J. 1996. Followers and outcasts: Berlin's Deaf community under national socialism, 1933–1945. *Collage* 33: 195–204.

Nagel, J. 1994. Constructing ethnicity: Creating and recreating ethnic identity and culture. *Social Problems* 41: 152–76.

National Association of the Deaf (NAD). 2000. *Cochlear implants: NAD position statement.* http://www.nad.org/site/pp.asp?c=foINKQMBFandb=138140.

National Inquiry into the Separation of Aboriginal and Torres Strait Islander Children from Their Families. 1997. *Bringing them home.* New South Wales, Australia: Sterling Press.

Newport, E. 1990. Maturational constraints on language learning. *Cognitive Science* 14: 11–28.

The New York Times. 1992. Deafness gene. February 18.

Nunes, R. 2001. Ethical dimensions of pediatric cochlear implantation. *Theoretical Medicine and Bioethics* 22: 337–49.

Padden C., and T. Humphries. 1988. *Deaf in America: Voices from a culture.* Cambridge Mass.: Harvard University Press.

Padden, C., and H. Markowicz. 1976. Cultural conflicts between hearing and deaf communities. In *VII World Congress of the World Federation of the Deaf,* ed. F. B. Crammatte and A. B. Crammatte, 407–11. Silver Spring Md.: National Association of the Deaf.

Padden, C., and C. Ramsey. 2000. American Sign Language and reading ability in Deaf children. In *Language acquisition by eye,* ed. C. Chamberlain, J. Morford, and R. Mayberry, 165–89. Mawah, N.J.: Erlbaum.

Peter, W. W. 1934. Germany's sterilization program. *American Journal of Public Health* 243: 187–91.

Petersen, W. 1980. Concepts of ethnicity. In *Harvard encyclopedia of American ethnic groups,* ed. S. Thernstrom, 234–42. Cambridge Mass.: Harvard University Press.

Petitto L. 1993. On the ontogenetic requirements for early language acquisition. In *Developmental neurocognition: Speech and face processing in the first year of life,* ed. E. de Boysson-Bardies, S. de Schonen, P. Jusczyk, and J. Morton, 365–83. New York, N.Y.: Kluwer Academic Press.

Ramsey, P. 1970. *The patient as person.* New Haven, Conn.: Yale University Press.

Reardon, W., H. Middleton-Price, S. Malcolm, P. Phelps, S. Bellman, L. Luxon, J. Martin, and A. Bumby. 1992. Clinical and genetic heterogeneity in X-linked deafness. *British Journal of Audiology* 26: 109–14.

Reefhuis, J., M. A. Honein, C. G. Whitney, S. Chamany, E. A. Mann, K. R. Biernath, K. Broder, et al. 2003. Risk of bacterial meningitis in children with cochlear implants. *New England Journal of Medicine* 349: 435–45.

Reisenberg, D., and R. M. Glass. 1989. The medical outcomes study. *Journal of the American Medical Association* 262: 943.

Saltus, R. 1989. Returning to the world of sound. *Boston Globe,* July 10, 27, 29.

Schein J. D. 1989. *At home among strangers.* Washington, D.C.: Gallaudet University Press.

Schneider, D. M. 1969. Kinship, nationality and religion in American culture: Toward a definition of kinship. In *Forms of symbolic action,* ed. R. F. Spencer, 116–25. Seattle, Wash.: University of Washington Press.

———. 1972. What is kinship all about? In *Kinship studies in the Morgan centennial year,* ed. P. Reining, 32–64. Washington, D.C.: Anthropological Society of Washington.

Schuchman, S,. and D. Ryan, eds. 2002. *Deaf people in Hitler's Europe.* Washington, D.C.: Gallaudet University Press.

Shapiro, J. P. 1993. *No pity: People with disabilities forging a new civil rights movement.* New York, N.Y.: Times Books.

Simon, R. J., and H. Altstein. 1992. *Adoption, race and identity: From infancy through adolescence.* New York, N.Y.: Praeger.

Smith, A. D. 1986. *The ethnic origin of nations.* Cambridge, United Kingdom: Blackwell.

Smith, S. 1995. Overview of genetic auditory syndromes. *Journal of the American Academy of Audiology* 6: 1–14.

Smith, T. 1997. Deaf people in context. Ph.D. diss., Anthropology Department, University of Washington, Seattle.

Sollors, W. 2001. Ethnic groups/ethnicity: Historical aspects. In *International encyclopedia of the social sciences*, ed. N. J. Smelser and P. B. Baltes, 4813–17. New York, N.Y.: Elsevier.

Strong, M., and P. Prinz. 1997. A study of the relationship between American Sign Language and English literacy. *Journal of Deaf Studies and Deaf Education* 2: 37–46.

Svirsky, M., S.-W. Teoh, and H. Neuburger. 2004. Development of language and speech perception in congenitally, profoundly deaf children as a function of age at cochlear implantation. *Audiology, Neuro-Otology* 9: 224–33.

Turnbull, C. M. 1962. *The forest people.* New York, N.Y.: Simon and Schuster.

Tye-Murray, N. 1992. *Cochlear implants and children: A handbook for parents, teachers and speech and hearing professionals.* Washington, D.C.: Alexander Graham Bell Association for the Deaf.

United Nations (UN). 1948. *Convention on the prevention and punishment of the crime of genocide: Resolution 96/I.* New York, N.Y.: United Nations.

———. 1992. *Declaration on the rights of persons belonging to national or ethnic, religious and linguistic minorities: Resolution 47/135.* New York, N.Y.: United Nations.

Valenstein, E. 1986. *Great and desperate cures.* New York: Basic Books.

Van Cleve, J., and B. Crouch. 1989. *A place of their own: Creating the deaf community in America.* Washington, D.C.: Gallaudet University Press.

Werth, B. 1991. How short is too short? *New York Times Magazine* (section 6), June 16, 14–17, 28–29, 47.

Winzer, M. A. 1986. Deaf-Mutia: Responses to alienation by the deaf in the mid-nineteenth century. *American Annals of the Deaf* 131: 29–32.

Zola, I. K. 1993. Disability statistics, what we count and what it tells us. *Journal of Disability Policy Studies* 4: 9–39.

4

PARENTS, CHILDREN, AND MEDICAL TREATMENT: LEGAL RIGHTS AND RESPONSIBILITIES

Eithne Mills

Mankind owes to the Child the best that it has to give . . .
—Geneva Declaration of the Rights of the Child, 1924

This chapter considers the nature and extent of the interaction that occurs between medicine and law whenever medical interventions are proposed. It does so in terms of the criterion of valid consent, which is the legal precondition that must be satisfied to protect the person's right to personal autonomy. An international search for legal cases in which the consent of a court has been sought in connection with cochlear implantation is analogous to the proverbial search for a needle in a haystack. Only one such case has been identified—a decision in the Federal Magistrates' Court of Australia. Although it is a decision of a court of summary jurisdiction only, and direction must first be gleaned from the established general precedents, the discussion therein does serve as a very useful pointer to the way in which other courts may lean in the future when faced, as they must inevitably be, with an action concerning the appropriateness of the implantation of a cochlear device into a child.

Consent to treatment is particularly complex when the recipient of medical care is a small child or adolescent. In recent decades, the question of a minor's competence to give or refuse consent was brought into sharp focus in the courts of various countries by way of contraception and sterilization matters, and it has more recently been considered in Australia in the context of sex affirmation procedures in children. Decisions made by the courts must necessarily derive from legal principle and may be made in reference to other cases in which legal precedent has been established.

Legal action in relation to medical intervention such as childhood cochlear implantation must be understood in relation to key legal doctrine, international convention, and established general precedent. This chapter begins with a discussion of notions of patriarchal power, the rights of the child established under international convention, and the principle of "best interests" in family law. The second part of the chapter introduces the legal notion of consent (in particular, what constitutes valid consent) and analyzes three cases of medical intervention in children. The first case to be discussed, *Secretary, Department of Health and Community Services v. JWB and Another* (Marion's case; 106 ALR 385), involving the sterilization of an intellectually impaired woman, established beyond doubt that a relevant Australian court can make virtually any order that is necessary to protect the welfare of children, providing that the court regards the best interests of the child as the paramount consideration. This power would clearly include implantation of a cochlear device and is therefore vital to an understanding of the issues involved in medical decision making by or on behalf of a child. The second case discussed, *Re Alex* (Hormonal Treatment for Gender Identity Dysphoria [2004] FamCA 297), raises fascinating questions in relation to the "best interests" principle and illustrates the Court's considerable respect for the young man involved. The final case, *L v. B*, is a parenting dispute involving issues of residence of and contact with a deaf baby as well as disagreement concerning medical treatment for the child, namely, cochlear implantation. It is with a view to considering the situation in that case of the child, D., and his parents that the legal principles and general precedents found in other cases of medical intervention of children are outlined earlier in the chapter.

LEGAL DOCTRINE AND PRINCIPLES

This section considers the evolving status of the child at law from "chattel" to bearer of considerable rights. It commences with a brief synopsis of early common law precepts of familial relationships, introduces the major children's human rights instruments of the twentieth century, and reviews the recent responses of both the Legislature and Judiciary to these developments in Australia.

Parents qua Guardians

The ancient doctrine of *patria potest* grounded Roman civil law, establishing the father as the head of the family. He held extensive powers and rights in relation to his wife and children, who were regarded as little more than his property, chattels over which he had an absolute right (Jones 1996). These notions of patriarchal power were carried over to the early common law by the doctrine of unity that denied any separate personhood to wives from their husbands. The doctrine similarly denied separate personhood to children from their fathers, at least until the children attained capacity by reaching their majority at the age of twenty-one years (Jones 1996).

In his famous "Commentaries," Blackstone (1765–1769) considered that "the power of parents over their children is derived from . . . their duty; this authority being given them, partly to enable the parent more effectually to perform his duty, and partly as a recompense for his care and trouble in the faithful discharge of it" (book 1, chap. 16). Although "Chancery, with its vague doctrine of *parens patriae*, and occasional interventions by ecclesiastical courts, accorded . . . slight amelioration of a paternalistic common law" (Foster 1974, 4), parental power over children was generally held in early case law to extend absolutely until the child's majority. It continued to do so until rejected a century later by Lord Denning, Master of the Rolls, who saw it as a dwindling authority that "starts with a right of control and ends with little more than advice" (*Hewer v. Bryant* [1970] 1 QB 369).

The age at which children now reach their majority is established by statute in all Australian states and territories as eighteen years. On attaining this age, they are considered to be adults, free of parental control and, absent of any impediments, able to make decisions as to their welfare entirely on their own behalf. Until that time, however, parents have decision-making obligations that exist to benefit their children, including making various medical decisions on their behalf, at least until they achieve capacity to make these decisions themselves.

Whether (and, if so, when) minors have sufficient cognition to consent to their own medical treatment, however, were questions long unanswered by the common law in Australia. Vexed by the prospect of arbitrarily imposed fixed limits on the process of "growing up," there was reluctance to impose artificiality and lack of realism in an area where the law must be sensitive (see Lord Scarman's comments, *Gillick v. West Norfolk Area Health Authority* [1986] AC 112, at [186]). As the New South Wales Law Reform Commission (NSW LRC) explained in a recent review of the relevant law, numerous studies of the capacity of young people to make their own decisions about their medical care now propose that the capacity to make an intelligent choice generally appears in a child between the ages of eleven and fourteen (NSW LRC 2004). The research also makes clear that young people's decision-making capacity must be judged according to their social development because the ability to make a free, deliberate choice is not simply dependant on cognitive maturity. There is, therefore, a risk of deferential responses to requests for consent being given until ages fifteen to seventeen years, associated with immaturity of judgment (NSW LRC 2004). According to the Commission, "The common law has developed a notion of consent arising out of an (adult) patient's right to self-determination or autonomy" (para. 1.38). This chapter seeks to explain how this position came about, how it affects those children whose physical development has followed a less common path, and what the corresponding obligations are of their parents and the medical professionals who treat them before they achieve decision-making capacity in their own right.

Establishing the Rights of the Child: An Early Declaration

The vulnerable nature of childhood was recognized in international instruments as early as 1924. In that year, the first *Declaration of the Rights of the Child* (the Geneva Declaration) was adopted by the League of Nations (1924). Thirty-five years later, in November 1959, the United Nations Geneva Assembly adopted the second *Declaration of the Rights of the Child* (United Nations 1959). The widespread acceptance of the idea that every individual, solely by virtue of being human, is entitled to enjoy human rights and freedoms is reflected in both the 1924 and 1959 instruments. It was not until the subsequent declaration in 1989, however, that voice was given to the concept of the best interests of the child being of primary importance.

The 1989 United Nations *Convention on the Rights of the Child* (the "UN Convention"; United Nations 1989) is premised on the fact that children have equal rights to respect. It recognizes them as participants in society in every aspect of their development and serves to protect their economic, social, cultural, civil, political, and humanitarian rights by the process of codification. A feature of the Convention is its suite of "guiding principles" that direct the way each right is to be fulfilled and respected. They serve as a constant reference for the implementation and monitoring of the rights of every child younger than the age of eighteen years, which are set out in the forty-one articles (paragraphs) of the Convention.

The UN Convention has been ratified by every country except the United States and Somalia. President Bill Clinton signed it during his office, but Congress has thus far failed to ratify it. Although the Convention was ratified by Australia in December 1990, it is yet to be incorporated fully into Australian law. The effect of Australia's international treaty obligations, however, was established by the majority of the High Court of Australia, which ruled the following:

> Ratification by Australia of an International Convention is not to be dismissed as merely a platitudinous or ineffectual act, particularly when the instrument evidences internationally accepted standards to be applied by courts and administrative authorities in dealing with basic human rights affecting the family and children. Rather, ratification of a Convention is a positive statement by the Executive Government of this country to the world and to the Australian people that the Executive Government and its agencies will act in accordance with the Convention. (*Minister of State for Immigration, Local Government and Ethnic Affairs v. Ah Hin Teogh* [1995] HCA 20[1995] 183 CLR 273[1995] 128 ALR 353 at [365])

The "Best Interests" Principle in Australian Family Law

A fundamental principle underlying the UN Convention is the "best interests of the child" (UN 1989, Article 3[1]), and this principle is reflected in the changes introduced in Australia under the *Family Law Reform Act 1995* (Commonwealth of Australia [Cth]). The Commonwealth of Australia is a federation of states each able to enact wide-ranging legislation in its own right very much the same as in the United States. The Commonwealth is only able to legislate where it is given power to do so under the Commonwealth Constitution. For example, the Constitution gives the Commonwealth plenary powers in relation to marriage and marital causes. Part VII, Division 10, of the Act provides that the "best interests of the child is the paramount consideration" for the parents and the court. Previously, under Australian law, the "welfare" of the child was the paramount consideration. Article 18 of the UN Convention endorses the concept of the best interests of the child and stipulates that parents share in the responsibility for the upbringing and development of their children. The UN Convention (UN 1989) recognizes, among others, the following rights: protection from all forms of violence (Article 19); special care and assistance where there is a disability (Article 23); the best available health care (Article 24); free public primary and appropriate secondary education so the child may develop her or his fullest human potential (Articles 28 and 29); and opportunities for leisure, recreation, and culture (Articles 30 and 31).

In an exercise of its powers under the Australian Constitution (Commonwealth of Australia Constitution Act [9 July 1900], ss51 [xxi] and [xxii]), the Parliament of the Commonwealth of Australia enacted the *Family Law Act 1975* (Cth) (the "FLA") and established the Family Court of Australia as the forum where issues relating to marriage, divorce, and matrimonial causes would be determined. The influence of the UN Convention is particularly evident in the statement of objectives in s60B of Part VII of the FLA, including under subsection (2c) that "parents share duties and responsibilities concerning the care, welfare and development of their children; and parents should agree about future parenting of their children."

Parents Have Responsibilities; Children Have Rights

The Family Court is a superior court of record and it is charged with ensuring that the best interests of the child are taken into account in arriving at decisions involving children (*Family Law Act 1975* [Cth], s65E). The prevailing message from the Full Court (in *Re B and B; Family Law Reform Act 1995* [1997] 21 Fam LR 676; FLC 92-755) was that, in Part VII cases, the essential inquiry is the best interest of the child. Decisions of the court in relation to children are known collectively as "parenting orders" (s64B[1]) and may deal with such matters as which person or persons with whom the child is to live, contact between a child and another person or persons, maintenance of a child, and any other aspect of parental responsibility for a child (including the provision of appropriate medical treatment) (s64B[2c]).

Section 61B of the FLA defines "parental responsibility" to mean "all the duties, powers, responsibilities and authority which, by law, parents have in relation to children." Section 61C stipulates that each parent of a child younger than the age of eighteen years has responsibility for that child. The notion of parental responsibility under Australian law, though having its origins in the United Kingdom's *Children's Act 1989,* can be distinguished from the latter in that it does not make reference to "parental rights." This change deliberately distances it from older terminologies suggestive of a proprietary relationship between parents and their children and thereby gives at least tacit recognition to children being possessed of the same rights to individual autonomy as adults.

LEGAL CONSENT TO MEDICAL INTERVENTION IN CHILDREN

A common precept of both the civil and criminal law in most, if not all, legal jurisdictions around the world is that conduct that constitutes an assault on, or a trespass to, the person is ordinarily unlawful. It is grounded in the notion that each person has a right to bodily integrity, that is, the right to choose what occurs in relation to their own person. As Blackstone (1765–1769) made clear,

> the law cannot draw the line between different degrees of violence, and therefore totally prohibits the first and lowest stage of it; every man's person being sacred, and no other having a right to meddle with it, in any the slightest manner. (120)

The law takes a holistic approach to the issue because

> human dignity requires that the whole personality be respected: the right to physical integrity is a condition of human dignity but the gravity of any invasion of physical integrity depends on its effect not only on the body but also upon the mind and on self-perception. (*Secretary, Department of Health and*

Community Services v. JWB and Another [Marion's case] High Court of Australia
[1992] HCA 15; [1992] CLR 218; F.C. 92/010 [6 May 1992])

Protection against an unauthorized invasion of the body and abuse of the fiduciary relationship of doctors toward patients is achieved by the process of "consent."[1] It is by way of consent that what would otherwise be unlawful contact may
be accepted, and therefore become acceptable in law. Although in most circumstances consensual contact is no longer regarded as an assault, there remain
exceptions to the rule of bodily inviolability. Sometimes consent may not be necessary to render the force lawful. That interpretation is of particular relevance to
a medical practitioner because he or she may escape liability where the intervention is a medical emergency and necessary to save the life or limb of a patient who
is unable to consent. At other times, irrespective of consent being given, it may
not be valid because the proposed intervention is not in the interests of the patient, the attendant risks are simply too great, or it is contrary to social policy. For
example, the surgical treatment of apotemnophilia, the desire to have a healthy
limb amputated, not only presents a major ethical issue for prospective surgeons
but also leaves them open to future actions in assault because its gravity is arguably beyond that to which a rational person can give his or her consent.

An understanding of these basic rules of law is of great importance to members of the medical profession because many medical and surgical procedures will
constitute an assault on the patient unless the patient has given prior consent. In
general terms, it means that before undertaking any intervention on the patient,
the practitioner must inform the patient of what is proposed and then obtain the
patient's permission to perform it. Many practitioners labor under the misappre-
hension that consent evidenced by a mere nod of the head or by even the signing
of a piece of paper is the end of the issue. True consent can be given only when
the rules of relevant disclosure have been satisfied.

The Essential Features of Valid Consent

For the consent to be effective and, if necessary, to withstand legal challenge, it
must be voluntary, and it must be made by a person of sound mind who is legally competent to consent. The practitioner must also at the least make sure that
the person giving the consent is "informed in broad terms of the nature of the
procedure that was intended" (*Chatterton v. Gerson and Another* [1981] QB 432 at
page 442 per Justice Bristow).

In Australia and the United Kingdom, the law has tended to differentiate
between the requirements necessary to vitiate an assault (consent) and those to
defend a charge of negligence (duty of disclosure). Although the paramount consideration is that people are entitled to make their own decisions about their lives
(*Rogers v. Whittaker* [1992] 175 CLR 479 at [487]), a prudent practitioner will make
sure not only to obtain the patient's consent to the procedure, but also to warn
them of any material risk inherent in a proposed procedure if

> a reasonable person in the patient's position, if warned of the risk, would be
> likely to attach significance to it or if the medical practitioner is or should

reasonably have been aware that the particular patient, if warned of the risk, would be likely to attach significance to it. (*Rogers v. Whittaker, para.* 490)

The patient must therefore be provided with, and understand, the "information which is material to the decision, especially as to the likely consequences of having or not having the treatment in question," irrespective of whether they ultimately consent or refuse to do so (*Re MB [Medical Treatment]* [1985] AC 871 per Lord Justice Butler-Sloss at [437]).

The doctrine of "informed consent" that has been developed in America is firmly rooted in the concept of a patient's rights and autonomy but is likewise seen as a protection against an unauthorized invasion of the body and abuse of the doctor-patient fiduciary relationship. Patients are regarded as having the decisive role in the medical decision-making process grounded in their constitutional right to self-determination (*Washington et al. v. Glucksberg et al.*, U.S. Supreme Court No. 96-110),[2] and the informed consent requirement is now enshrined in law throughout the United States. Australian courts have tended to be dismissive of the "informed consent" terminology (see *Rogers v. Whittaker* [1992] 175 CLR 479 at [490]) in adult cases but have progressively moved to adopt the broad concept, especially in cases involving children.

Consent to Medical Treatment for Children

As was stated above, the Family Court of Australia is a creature of the Commonwealth and was established by the *Family Law Act 1975.* Amendments to the Act in 1983 served to expand the Court's jurisdiction concerning children in a number of ways, including the permitting of proceedings that concerned the protection of the welfare of a child of a marriage, thus "investing courts exercising jurisdiction under the Act with (exclusive) power similar to the wardship power of the State Supreme Courts" (Evans 1983, 1097).

The original jurisdiction encompassed only children of de jure marriages but was subsequently extended in Australia by the *Family Law Amendment Act 1987* (Cth) to include children of all relationships. This extension was made possible by the referral from the states to the Commonwealth of their powers in respect to guardianship, custody, maintenance, and access in relation to exnuptial children. The states, however, still retain jurisdiction to deal with adoption (except in Victoria) and state-level child welfare matters.

The Australian *Family Law Reform Act 1995* (Cth) introduced the concept of "parenting orders," which are orders to be made with respect to the best interests of the child as the paramount consideration (Section 65E). These orders confer on a person the parental responsibility for a child, but only to the extent that the order confers duties, powers, responsibilities, or authority in relation to the child. Making a decision as to what may truly be in the best interests of a child, however, is not always simple, as is illustrated by the following discussion.

Three cases are described and analyzed here to illustrate the legal principles involved and general precedents established in the area of consent to medical intervention of children. The first, which has become widely known as *Marion's* case[3] ([1990] 14 Fam LR 427), was first referred to the Full Court of the Family

Court for determination and was subsequently appealed to the High Court ([1992] HCA 15). It deals with sterilization by way of surgical procedure. The second case discussed is *Re Alex* ([2004] FamCA 297), which deals with hormonal treatment for gender identity dysphoria. The final case, *L v. B*, which deals with the court's ability to order cochlear implantation, was heard by the Family Court in 2004 and was influenced by the first two cases.

Marion's Case

In 1990, the Full Court of the Family Court was called on to consider whether the parents, as guardians of their daughter, then at the age of thirteen years, could authorize her sterilization by way of a surgical procedure without an order of the Court. The daughter, Marion, suffered considerable intellectual and physical impairment and was consequently incapable of caring for herself or properly understanding the nature and implications of sexuality and motherhood. The application first came before Chief Justice Nicholson, and he determined to state a case for the opinion of the Full Court as to questions of law arising out of the application. The Full Court held, inter alia, with Justices Strauss and McCall, with Chief Justice Nicholson dissenting, that the parents could make the decision without its sanction ([1990] 14 FamLR 427). The Northern Territory Department of Health and Community Services appealed the answers given by the Full Court to the High Court.

The parents argued before the High Court that the decision to sterilize their child was not significantly different from other major decisions that parents are required to make on behalf of their children and, therefore, the involvement of the Family Court was optional and of a supervisory nature only. The majority, Chief Justice Mason and Justices Dawson, Toohey, and Gaudron, however, agreed with the submission of the appellant Northern Territory Department, being also the opinion of Chief Justice Nicholson at first instance. It held that the parents as guardians could not authorize sterilization of a child without the consent of the Family Court other than in exceptional circumstances such as where it was incidental to the treatment of a life-threatening illness (*Marion's* case 106 ALR 385, page 26). The majority also held that proceedings concerning the welfare of a child of a marriage that involve at least one of the parties to the marriage are an exclusive matter for the Family Court (para. 28). The power of the Court to make orders in relation thereto is only subject to the limitation that an order cannot be made in relation to a child who is in the custody of, or under the guardianship, care and control or supervision of, a person under a child welfare law (*Family Law Act 1975* [Cth], s60H[1]). To arrive at its decision, the High Court carefully considered two issues of substantial importance in cases involving children, the doctrine of "informed consent" and the "welfare" or *parens patriae* jurisdiction of the Family Court.

In *Marion's* case (106 ALR 385), all members of the High Court emphasized the fundamental right to personal inviolability that exists in common law. This right underscores the principles of criminal and civil assault as well as the need to determine the individual's consent to surrender that right (*Marion's* case 106 ALR 385, page 26). The threshold question of consent in this particular case was whether any child, intellectually disabled or not, is capable, in law or in fact, of consenting to medical treatment on his or her own behalf. It should be noted that the Court did not actually define the term *informed consent*. However, following the ratio established by the House of Lords in *Gillick v. West Norfolk Area Health Authority* [1986] AC 112, it endorsed a test under which a young person's competence to consent to medical treatment was assessed according to his or her ability to understand the nature and consequences of the proposed treatment. The proposition endorsed by the majority in *Gillick* was that parental power to consent to medical treatment on behalf of a child diminishes gradually as the child's capacities and maturity grow and that this rate of development depends on the individual child (*Marion's* case 106 ALR 385, page 12). In the words of the Court, a minor is capable of giving informed consent when he or she "achieves a sufficient understanding and intelligence to enable him or her to understand fully what is proposed" (*Marion's* case, 106 ALR 385, page 3). The test had elements of both (a) the notion of consent as an agreement to what would otherwise be an unlawful trespass of the individual and (b) a decision made pursuant to the disclosure of all material risks. It removed much of the previous uncertainty of the common law of Australia as to whether minors younger than sixteen years can ever consent to medical treatment, recognizing that there is, in ordinary circumstances, a steady ascendancy of the child's autonomous decision-making rights and a corresponding decline in the associated rights (and duty) of the child's parents to make decisions on the child's behalf in the years leading up to the age of majority (*Marion's* case, 106 ALR 385, page 12). The majority decision of the Court in *Marion's* case also made very plain that

> it cannot be presumed that an intellectually disabled child is, by virtue of his or her disability, incapable of giving consent to treatment. The capacity of a child to give informed consent to medical treatment depends on the rate of development of each individual. (14)

The child in the case was factually incapable of consenting to medical treatment; thus, the second question requiring an answer from the Court was whether the proposed treatment was within the scope of the parental power to give consent on behalf of their child. The question necessarily concerned the limits of parental power other than limits arising from the child's incapacity to give her personal consent. Where incapacity arises as a consequence of the child's minority, responsibility for the decisions is ordinarily vested in the minor's parent or other guardian who may, in a wide range of circumstances, consent to medical treatment of their child who is a minor. The Court noted that "parental consent, when effective, is itself an exception to the need for personal consent to medical treatment" (*Marion's* case 106 ALR 385, page 10) and that, where the power exists, "the overriding criterion to be applied in its exercise is the welfare of the child objectively assessed" (14). Authority to consent to the sterilization of a child, however, was regarded by the majority as a special case.

After looking at the Australian case law on the issue and making comparisons with decisions in other common law jurisdictions, the majority found that there are features involved in a decision to authorize sterilization such that, to best protect the child's interests, it should not come within the ordinary scope of parental power to consent to it; court authorization is necessary as a procedural safeguard (*Marion's* case 106 ALR 385, page 23). Although it hesitated to use terms such as *therapeutic* and *nontherapeutic*, the Court said such a distinction was necessary given that the context in which the Court was considering was sterilization. That is, the case did not include sterilization as a secondary consequence of surgery appropriately carried out to treat some malfunction or disease (*Marion's* case 106 ALR 385, page 23). The decision was justified, according to the Court, by factors that include the major, invasive, and irreversible nature of the procedure; the significant risk of making the wrong decision as to either a child's present or future capacity to consent or the best interests of a child who cannot consent; and the gravity of the consequences of a wrong decision (23). The majority concluded that

> the gravity of wrongly authorising [surgery] flows both from the resulting inability to reproduce and from the fact of being acted upon contrary to one's wishes or best interests. The fact of violation is likely to have social and psychological implications concerning the person's sense of identity, social place and self-esteem. (*Marion's* case 106 ALR 385, page 25)

Insofar as the power of the Family Court to make consent decisions with respect to medical treatment of minors was concerned, the majority said that the 1983 amendments to the *Family Law Act 1975* vested in the Family Court the substance of the *parens patriae* jurisdiction (*Marion's* case 106 ALR 385, page 30). Historically, *parens patriae* belonged to the King who, as parent of the country, had responsibility for the care of those who were not able to take care of themselves. According to Justice La Forest in *Re Eve* ([1986] 2 SCR, at 407–417; [1986] 31 DLR [4th], at 14–21), "the Crown has an inherent jurisdiction to do what is for the benefit of the incompetent. Its limits have not, and cannot be defined" (*Re Eve*, para. 31). The majority in *Marion's* case likewise found that more contemporary descriptions of this inherent jurisdiction invariably accept that there is no limitation on it except that it must be exercised in accordance with principle. The Family Court can therefore authorize sterilization of a child because it "can exercise jurisdiction in cases where parents have no power to consent to an operation, as well as cases in which they have the power" (*Marion's* case 106 ALR 385, page 385). The Appeals Court of the Supreme Court of New South Wales similarly considered that "where it is lawful for an adult to obtain a medical procedure, it is legitimate for a court in the exercise of its *parens patriae* jurisdiction to consent on behalf of a child" (*K v. Minister for Youth and Community Services* [1982] 1 NSWLR 311). Chief Justice Nicholson subsequently handed down a decision in those terms in the originating case in the Family Court (*Re Marion* [No.2] [1992] 17 Fam LR 336).

The Case of *P v. P*

The importance of assessing all alternative avenues of treatment before undertaking a surgical intervention was considered also in *P v. P* ([1995] FLC 92-615; [1994] 181 CLR 583), a further case involving the sterilization of an intellectually impaired young woman. The High Court drew attention in *Marion's* case to the possibility of inconsistencies between the *parens patriae* jurisdiction given to the Family Court by Part VII of the Family Law Act 1975 (Cth) and the jurisdiction granted to various creatures of state legislation. These differences in jurisdiction, however, were unexplored as Their Honors were not then called on to determine such issues with reference to the Children (Care and Protection) Act 1987 (NSW) (*Marion's* case 106 ALR 385, page 35). They were considered by the High Court subsequently, however, in the matter of *P v. P* ([1994] HCA 20; [1994] CLR 583; [1994] 120 ALR 545).

In *P v. P*, the young person, who was intellectually impaired and also suffered from epilepsy, lived in New South Wales. The legislation in that state permitted only the Guardianship Board to authorize sterilization surgery to save her life or prevent serious damage to her health. No such authorization was given. Her parents therefore applied to the Family Court for authorization to prevent her menstruating or becoming pregnant. On appeal, a majority of the High Court (Chief Justice Mason as well as Justices Deane, Toohey, and Gaudron) held that the Family Court's jurisdiction prevailed over that of the New South Wales Board (and by implication any similar Board that was empowered to make a comparable decision). [Justice] McHugh . . . agreed as to the general effect but expressed further views because, as Nicholson, Harrison, and Sandor (1996) explained some years later,

> the Family Court's jurisdiction prevails as a consequence of s109 of the Constitution. That section resolves inconsistencies between State and Commonwealth power in favour of the Commonwealth. McHugh J departed from the majority on this aspect as his Honour did not characterise the proceedings before the Board as proceedings in a Court and considered that it was the making of an order which attracted the operation of s109 of the Constitution. (242)

Possibly the most important aspect of the Full Court's findings in *P v. P*, however, was its discussion of the proper approach to the "step of last resort" test laid down in *Marion's* case where the majority said that "in the context of medical management, it is a convenient way of saying that alternative and less invasive procedures have all failed or that it is certain that no other procedure or treatment will work" (*Marion's* case 106 ALR 385, page 32). In *P v. P*, the High Court rejected the approach of the trial judge who had applied a version of the "but for test." The trial judge did this test by comparing the young woman's circumstances with those of a hypothetical young woman who did not have the particular disabilities on the premise that "sterilisation should not be approved if it would not be contemplated in the case of an intellectually normal girl with similar epilepsy" (*P v. P* [1994] 181 CLR 583, at 82 and 146). The Full Court of the High Court held that such an approach might distract a court from its fundamental task of deciding whether, in a particular case, citing the majority in *Marion's* case, "a [sterilisation] procedure is necessary to enable her to lead a life in keeping with her own needs and capacities" (*Marion's* case, 106 ALR 385, page 32).

In a wide ranging discussion, Nicholson, Harrison, and Sandor (1996, 105) subsequently stated that they read the majority's reference to determining whether a procedure is a step of last resort "in the context of a child's needs and capacities, [as] requiring an appreciation of the interaction of that child's abilities and disabilities when considering the proposed treatment."

The Case of *Re Alex*

The very recent case of *Re Alex* (Hormonal Treatment for Gender Identity Dysphoria) [2004] FamCA 297) was an application before Chief Justice Nicholson in the Family Court by a state child welfare department on behalf of an adolescent seeking medical treatment for transsexualism (see also Mills 2004, 2005). Alex, who was under a child welfare order issued by the relevant state, was a thirteen year old with female phenotype and genotype who had a long and consistent history of asserting that he was a male and taking all possible steps to project a male sexual identity both at home and at school. There was no evidence of any contradicting psychopathology, and there ensued a consensus diagnosis of gender identity disorder consistent with transsexualism. Alex was revealed to be suffering concurrent severe frustration and depression accompanied by suicidal ideations as a consequence of his inner conflict and his inability to resolve it thus far. Orders were sought that would allow him to commence hormonal treatment as the first step toward affirming his sexual identity as a male; the application before the Court did not contemplate any surgical procedures being performed before Alex would attain the age of eighteen years (*Re Alex* [2004] FamCA 297, para. 2). Although all the evidence before the Court supported hormonal intervention as being in Alex's best interests, there was some divergence of opinion as to its precise course and timing (para. 5).

The Chief Justice commenced his judgment by stating the basis of the Court's jurisdiction in the matter. He identified two important considerations going to the question that arose from the High Court's decision in *Marion's* case: whether the child or young person is himself competent to consent and whether the subject matter of the application is a "special medical procedure" to which a parent or guardian cannot consent (*Marion's* case 106 ALR 385, page 152). The gravamen of the decision in that case, as extracted by His Honor, was that "if a child or young person cannot consent her/himself to a medical procedure, parental consent (which for present purposes may be equated with that of a guardian) is ineffective where the proposed intervention is: invasive, permanent and irreversible; and not for the purpose of curing a malfunction or disease" (*Marion's* case 106 ALR 385, page 153).

Considering whether the treatment proposed for Alex constituted a special medical procedure, His Honor reviewed several other decisions where the Court had exercised its welfare jurisdiction in relation to procedures other than sterilization and likewise found that jurisdiction extended beyond the single issue of sterilization considered in *Marion's* case. In particular, he referred to a passage in *Re GWW and CMW* ([1997] FLC 92-748) where Justice Hannon, facing a challenge to the Court's jurisdiction, cited the High Court's decision in *Marion's* case where it found at page 23 that court authorization was required because of the significant risk of making a wrong decision and the particularly grave consequences of such a decision (*Re GWW and CMW*, para. 176). His Honor agreed with what he saw as Justice Hannon's conclusion that the welfare jurisdiction was not limited to cases involving only surgical intervention (*Re GWW and CMW*, para. 178). His Honor, however, then distinguished the present case from *Re GWW and CMW* where an application for approval to harvest stem cells from the child for the benefit of another family member was refused on the basis that the procedure was not in the child's best interests and where the proposed procedures in *Re Alex* were, in fact, in the best interest of Alex.

The Cochlear Implantation Case of *L v. B*

It was not until very recently that an Australian court was asked to consider whether it had power to order cochlear implantation on the application of one parent. The matter of *L v. B* ([2005] 185 FLR 305, 32 Fam LR 169, [2004] FMCAfam 312) was a parenting dispute involving issues of residence and contact. There was also a disagreement concerning medical treatment for the child D. who was the only child of a short relationship between the applicant mother and the respondent father. D. was eighteen months old at the time of the application and profoundly deaf (with Waardenburg Syndrome). For approximately thirteen months before the hearing date, D. lived predominantly with his mother. During that period, his father had contact with D. from 9:00 a.m. to 4:00 p.m. on three days of each week. Both parents were also profoundly deaf since birth.

The orders sought from the Family Court related to residence, contact, and the specific issue of medical treatment. In the context of the specific issues order, D.'s mother applied to the Court seeking authorization of a proposed medical intervention involving the implant of a cochlear device. The Court noted that at the heart of this dispute about medical treatment were the different views of the mother and father about how D. should be raised as a deaf child in a mainly hearing world.

The Evidence of the Parents

The crux of the father's disagreement with cochlear implantation of D. was that deafness is not a disability that needed to be fixed by an operation to make him hear. The father also argued that D. could grow into a happy and independent adult by learning signed language and other ways of communicating in the deaf community. The father also argued that the medical treatment would make contact between father and son more difficult in the future.

In evidence, the Court heard that the father has been profoundly deaf since birth and, in common with D., has Waardenburg Syndrome. The father had, however, by the use of hearing aids, experienced a significant improvement in "aural awareness" that enabled him to "hear D. laugh, dogs barking and trucks approaching" (*L v. B* [2004] FMCAfam 312, para. 32). The Court also heard evidence of the father's participation in many sporting activities and his concern that a cochlear implant would prevent D. from similar enjoyment. It was obvious from his evidence that D.'s father strongly identified with Deaf culture and agreed with the view that after being fitted with hearing aids or cochlear implants, hearing impaired children "often do not receive enough support and information to cope with their deafness" (a view initially expressed by a witness, "R.W.," who was a full-time community worker for the Queensland Deaf Society). He also agreed with the assertion that "culturally deaf children (children who identify with the deaf community) are automatically placed in schools that have deaf units where all their needs are usually met" (*L v. B*, para. 23).

D.'s mother was equally strong in her view that D. should have the opportunity to move freely not only in the hearing community but also in the Deaf community. She argued that cochlear implantation would help him achieve this freedom. Although she was eager that D. should receive a cochlear implant as soon as practicable, it was, from her evidence, apparent that D.'s mother was mindful of the benefits flowing from the use of signing. Federal Magistrate Baumann stated:

I am satisfied that the mother understands that it is imperative that D. also learn to sign. I noticed in Court that although it appeared the mother could effectively lip read, she relied substantially on the sign interpreters provided to the Court. The mother says that 90 percent of her friends are deaf and she communicates with them by signing. (*L v. B*, para. 15)

The mother gave evidence of having been profoundly deaf since birth, but now, with the use of hearing aids, she has 10 percent capacity to hear. Both her parents are hearing, and she stated her intention to seek cochlear implantation surgery for herself in the future. Speaking of her own experience and her wishes for D., she said:

I have experienced first hand the difficulties and frustrations of being deaf in a hearing community. I have difficulty communicating with hearing people, difficulty making myself understood at times even though in the deaf community I am considered to have a high level of speech. I am fully aware of the fact that D. will always have to move in both deaf and hearing communities as both his father and myself [sic] are deaf. I would wish for D. to also be able to move freely in the hearing community and be able to experience the opportunities I have not have [sic] for learning and communication. I feel that it is in D.'s best interest to have the surgery now and should he as an adult choose not to use the implant he can at least make an informed choice of what he wants to do. (*L v. B*, para. 13)

Both the mother and the father had separate legal representation, as did D. The purpose of providing a child with separate representation was described as ensuring that the Court has all relevant evidence available when it comes to adjudicate the matter in dispute and that the child has a voice in proceedings (*Re K* [1994] 17 Fam LR 537).

The Medical Evidence: How the Court Informed Itself

Integral to the giving of valid consent to a medical procedure is the entitlement to information before consent. In other words, a patient is entitled to be informed about the nature and risks of a proposed treatment. Equally, the Family Court, before giving consent to medical treatment of a minor, must be satisfied that it has sufficient information on which to base a valid consent to a decision that reflects the best interests of the child in question. The relevant information is normally furnished to the Court by way of the opinion of an expert in a particular relevant field. An expert's opinion is admissible to furnish the Court with scientific information that is likely to be outside the knowledge and experience of a judge and jury (*R v. Turner* [1975] QB 834 at 841; Approved, *Murphy v. R* [1989] 167 CLR 94 at 111). Either party to a proceeding before a court may obtain an expert's report from a person with the appropriate expertise.

In *L v. B*, the Court heard evidence from medical practitioners who were experts in otolaryngology, from various speech pathologists and audiologists, and from a psychologist[4] who provided a report on the family. The Court placed major reliance on the evidence of the three otolaryngologists called on behalf of the mother, which Federal Magistrate Baumann referred to as "unchallenged and of high quality" (*L v. B* [2004] FMCAfam 312, para. 28). The respondent father did not rely on any direct medical evidence from medical practitioners, but relied solely on the evidence of a speech pathologist and audiologist. Federal Magistrate Baumann made clear that he recognized the vital importance of D. learning signing to "not only ensure effective communication with his father, but also the wider deaf community of which he is a member" ([2004] FMCAfam 312, para. 35). Such a course was endorsed by Dr. Parker and Professor Gibson although not favored by Professor Black, the medical director of the Hear and Say Centre.

Just as His Honor recognized the importance of D. learning to communicate by signing, he was also respectful of Deaf culture, stating that it "was clear to me that the unusual circumstances of this case have created a fertile environment for the advocates of what appears to be a live issue in the deaf community to have their say" ([2004] FMCAfam 312, para. 37).

He referred to Professor Gibson's observations that

> deaf people have developed their own method of communicating using sign. To many deaf people, speech is unnecessary as they feel they can achieve everything they wish to using sign. Sign has become a normal means of communication for them and they have developed their own deaf culture or society. Many deaf people feel that a cochlear implant is an attempt by hearing people to make deaf people into hearing people taking them away from their own deaf culture. ([2004] FMCAfam 312, para. 32)

The Court's Decision to Authorize the Procedure

The Court concluded that the matter before it was a medical procedure application within the meaning of Division 4.2.3 of the *Family Law Amendment Rules 2004* (Cth), being a "major medical procedure designed to treat a bodily malfunction"—namely D.'s deafness (*L v. B*, [2004] FMCAfam 312, para. 10). Granting residence to the mother with interim contact with the father and approving the mother's application for medical treatment of the child D., Federal Magistrate Baumann held that

> the medical evidence was that D. was a suitable recipient for a cochlear implant and that it should be performed before the child was 2–2½ years old. The optimal opportunity to derive the maximum benefits from the surgery and resultant post-surgery therapy would occur if the surgery occurred forthwith. ([2004] FMCAfam 312, para. 51)

The effect of the medical evidence was that it was considered in D.'s best interest that he receive the implant as soon as practicable so as to maximize his ability to be bilingual, to have a "normal-sounding" voice, to achieve educationally in the future, and to interact in the predominantly hearing world in which he lives. Ultimately, the Court considered the best interests of the child were served by giving him the necessary foundations at an early developmental stage of his life, on which he could build the skills, strengths, and understanding to reach his potential as an adult. The decision was not intended to give validity, as a superior approach or view, to either side in the debate over childhood cochlear implantation that engulfs the Deaf community. The orders represented what was in the best interests of the child, according to the evidence at the time, and that was the paramount consideration.

WHERE LIES THE FUTURE?

Today, parents in Australia who are guardians of a deaf child, where they are in agreement that the interests of that child are best served by resort to cochlear implant surgery, have prima facie authority to give their valid consent to such a procedure. This authority is predicated on the view that the surgery, while fitting the criterion of a major medical procedure, is designed to treat a "bodily malfunction" (the child's deafness) and therefore falls outside the special category of procedures contemplated by Division 4.2.3 of the *Family Law Rules 2004* (Cth). Its validity therefore relies on the view currently prevailing among medical experts and consequently accepted by the courts that deafness *is* a bodily malfunction.

A question less clear, and even more sensitive in this context, is whether a child who feels harmed by *failure* to implant may sue a parent for damages. Parents and medical practitioners should be aware that, even though this issue is very much a developing jurispridence and matters of law are complicated by difficult issues of policy, such an action is a possibility. Although it is outside the scope of this chapter to discuss the question in depth, some coverage of this issue is therefore necessary.

At common law there existed between husband and wife immunity from suit in tort that has now largely been abolished by statute. Some American courts extended interfamilial immunity to actions between parent and child, but this approach has never been part of Australian law. Simply, it is not beyond the bounds of possibility that children may sue the surgeon for negligence, and duty of care proceedings may one day be instituted against a parent (or parents) for failing to follow medical recommendations that cochlear implantation of their child should be performed. In the case of an omission, the harm is brought about by a person's failure to act rather than a person's engagement in an action that inflicts harm.

There is a distinction at law between liability for acts performed in a negligent manner and liability for omissions. Where positive actions result in the infliction of harm, negligence may be found if the harm was reasonably foreseeable. Courts are mindful that rendering a person liable for an omission, however, involves imposing a duty on them to act, which may be viewed as an interference with personal liberties. Although the courts are therefore often reluctant to sanction such liability for an omission solely on the basis of the foreseeability of harm, it may be that a future decision will consider the UN Convention's exhortations with respect to the rights of children to be compelling. Therefore, the existence and scope of a parent's duty may be extended to include a duty to explore all medical and therapeutic avenues open to the parent to enhance the welfare of a child.

Notes

1. A fiduciary relationship is one of trust and confidence (*Boardman v. Phipps* [1967] 2 AC 46). It gives the fiduciary, who has a duty to act in good faith for the benefit of the other, a special opportunity to exercise a power to the detriment of that other person who is accordingly vulnerable to abuse by the fiduciary of his or her position (*Hospital Products Ltd. v. United States Surgical Corporation* [1984] 156 CLR 41; 55 ALR 417).
2. Argued January 8, 1997; decided June 26, 1997; see also *Schloendorff v. Society of New York Hospital*, 21 N.Y. 125, 129, 105 N.E. 92, 93 (1914); *Cruzan v. Director, Mo. Dept. of Health*, 497 U.S. Supreme Court at 269–279.
3. *Secretary, Department of Health and Community Services v. JWB and Anor* (*Marion's* case) 106 A.L.R. 385; [1992] HCA 15; (1992) CLR 218; F.C. 92/010 (6 May 1992).
4. Dr. Bruce Black (professor of otolaryngology at the University of Queensland); Dr. Anthony Parker (head of Auditory Rehabilitation and Cochlear Implant Services, Mater Hospital); Professor William Gibson (director of the Cochlear Implant Centre, New South Wales, and professor of otolaryngology at University of Sydney); Mr. Ronald Morris (speech therapist) and Ms. Sharon Ewing (audiologist) for the father; Ms. Karen McGhie (audiologist), Ms. Sue Hodgman (speech pathologist), and Mr. Lassig (speech therapist) for the mother; Ms. Denise Britton (psychologist).

References

Blackstone, W. 1765–1769. Of parent and child. In *Commentaries on the laws of England*, book 1, chapter 16, http://www.yale.edu/lawweb/avalon/blackstone/blacksto.htm.

Evans, G. J. 1983. *Second reading of the Family Law Amendment bill 1983*. Senate Hansard, June 1, 1983.

Foster, H. H. 1974. A "bill of rights" for children. Springfield, Ill.: Thomas.

Jones, M. 1996. Mediating rights: Children, parents and the state. *Australian Journal of Human Rights* 2: 2.

League of Nations. 1924. Geneva Declaration of the Rights of the Child of 1924, *adopted* Sept. 26, 1924, O.J. Spec. Supp. 21, at 43.

Mills, E. 2004. Re Alex: Adolescent gender identity disorder and the Family Court of Australia. *Deakin Law Review* 9 (2):365–73.

———. 2005. A question of gender: Re Alex, adolescent gender identity disorder and the Family Court. *Law Institute Journal* 79 (3):38.

New South Wales Law Reform Commission. 2004. Issues paper 24: Minor's consent to medical treatment. Sydney: New South Wales Law Reform Commission. Available at http://www.lawlink.nsw.gov.au/lrc.nsf/pages/ip24chp01#.

Nicholson, A., M. Harrison, and D. Sandor. 1996. The role of the family court in medical procedure cases. *Australian Journal of Human Rights* 2 (2):242.

United Nations. 1959. Declaration of the rights of the child (1959). General Assembly resolution.
1386(XIV), November 20. 14 U.N. GAOR Supp. (No. 16) at 19.
———. 1989. Convention on the rights of the child. UN General Assembly document A/RES/44/2, December 12.

5

MEDIA REPRESENTATION AND COCHLEAR IMPLANTATION

Linda Komesaroff

The daily press has been reporting on cochlear implantation for more than two decades. In doing so, it has not only reflected but also shaped the representations of deafness as well as constructed particular views of deaf people and cochlear implantation. Deaf people have sought access to and inclusion in the media and have, at times, successfully engaged in "textual relationships of power" (Luke 2000, 449). This chapter draws on a comprehensive analysis of media articles to show how key issues related to implantation have been represented to the public.

An analysis of media representation provides insight into how power works in society and the ways in which the media is implicated in maintaining inequalities. For example, textual analysis of media articles on cochlear implantation has identified the way in which particular versions of reality are constructed and how readers are positioned in relation to that world (Komesaroff 2002). An analysis of the representation of deafness in the Australian press from 1982 to 2003 identified the dominance of the medical-disability model of deafness over the "sociocultural" model in articles related to childhood implantation (Power 2005).

The study reported in this chapter extends the scope and focus of this type of analysis to articles on cochlear implantation published since 1982. The newspaper databases Factiva and Newsbank were searched for the term *cochlear* in all regions of the world. The earliest article located was published in 1982, and the search identified more than 7,000 articles on Factiva alone; the search term *cochlear implant* yielded 2,426 articles. Given the significantly reduced number of articles located with this latter term, the broader term *cochlear* was used and irrelevant articles were removed manually. Articles that related only to financial reviews, listings on the stock exchange, and contract tenders or articles that did not relate to cochlear implantation were identified on the basis of headline and lead paragraph. Multiple listings of articles within or across both databases were also removed manually.

The search resulted in slightly more than a hundred articles identified from the 1980s, hundreds from the 1990s, and thousands from the 2000s (on average, more than 1,000 articles have been published each year since 2000). The first stage of the study, reported in this chapter, includes an analysis of all relevant articles identified from the period of the 1980s, totaling 114 articles. Further articles published since the early 1990s were selected on the basis of searches done on keywords related to issues or themes that arose during the study (including terms such as *meningitis, implant-related deaths* and use of particular language such as *miracle cure*). Most articles indexed in the databases were published in the United

88

States, Australia, and the United Kingdom, which is unsurprising given the United States and Australian origins of cochlear implant developers: Dr. William House, the U.S. otologist who produced the first wearable single-channel implant in 1969, and Professor Graeme Clark, who pioneered the multichannel cochlear implant, the first device implanted in 1978.

Through a process of grounded theory (that is, starting with empirical data without preconceived theories), key categories were identified from the hundreds of articles analyzed in this study (categories such as "expectations," "reported outcomes," "historical events"; further subcategories were identified, including "expectations of parents" and "expectations of professionals"). Sections of text were tagged according to the identified categories and the themes that emerged during the analysis. This process often required multiple readings of the text and the recoding of articles as key categories were identified and clarified. The focus of data analysis was on the anticipated benefits of implantation, the reported outcomes of implantation (anecdotal and science-based), the shifting criteria for implantation, technological developments, financial imperatives, and the representation of deafness and the response by Deaf people.

The results presented in this chapter primarily focus on the first decade of media reports, with some reference made to more recent articles where relevant. This focus enables an historical account of implantation and allows one to view the outcomes of implantation (reported at the time) with the benefit of hindsight. That is, the claims made of implantation when it first became publicly available and gained U.S. Food and Drug Administration (FDA) approval can be contrasted with later reports of actual accounts from implant recipients, their parents, and cochlear implant professionals.

It is also instructive to review the path taken by a multibillion dollar industry (world leader Cochlear Corporation reporting sales revenues over the past decade of nearly 2 billion dollars) and one that, worldwide, has gained access to millions of research dollars and philanthropic donations (Cochlear's Research and Development expenditure from 1996 to 2005 has been more than 258 million dollars). The industry has also gained FDA approval with what some say was limited evidence of success, and it has continued to thrive despite more recent reports of deaths from meningitis linked to a U.S. implant device (*Wall Street Journal* 2002), a criminal investigation by the U.S. Department of Justice into the relationship between Cochlear's American subsidiary and doctors, the subsequent resignation of the head of North American operations, the 18 percent plummet its shares took to a four-year low (Mcadam and Eyers 2004), and the continued opposition from Deaf communities and their leaders (*The Observer*). Investors in Cochlear and other manufacturers (including boards of directors, senior executives, and others whose remuneration is linked to the company's success) have stood to make enormous financial gain. Cochlear's share prices, for example, made a ten-year leap from $3.40 in 1996 to a reported $39.20 at the end of the 2005 financial year (Cochlear 2005).

THE ANTICIPATED BENEFITS OF IMPLANTATION

The earliest identified press article about cochlear implantation, published by *The Globe and Mail* in Vancouver in 1982 (Rabkin 1982), reported the implantation of the first Canadian adult. It was reported that cochlear implantation was "supposed to enable a profoundly deaf person to recapture some hearing" (13). When the FDA approved the cochlear implant for use on an experimental basis with adults two years later, in November 1984, it was reported that "an electronic ear implant . . . could enable 60,000 to 200,000 profoundly deaf people in the United States to hear sounds such as automobile horns and door bells" (Molotsky 1984, 1). Within one or two years, U.S. press articles were heralding the end to deafness or making extraordinary claims such as the following:

> These are doctors who can make the stone deaf hear music and follow conversations, word by word. . . . [It is] a bionic hearing device that has conquered deafness in more than 200 men, women and children worldwide . . . [and] may enable doctors to virtually *cure deafness* in hundreds of cases. (*The Seattle Times* 1985, 14, emphasis added)

* * *

> More advancements are coming, including one which might make total deafness obsolete. . . . "This kind of product has the ability to make a totally deaf person hear," Mr. Tucker [president, R.P. Scherer Corporation] says. (Shaw 1985, 98)

* * *

> It brings hearing to children who are either born deaf or developed hearing impairments from meningitis or other illnesses. (Ricks 1986, 1)

* * *

> Doctors have implanted a fascinating new device into the ear of a San Diego resident, restoring to a major extent that person's ability to hear normally after years of total deafness. (Smollar 1986, 5)

* * *

> "This new device is fascinating in that *you can have a person talking normally three weeks later.*" (Dr. Terence Davidson of the University of California San Diego Center's Head and Neck Surgery Division, cited in Smollar 1986, 5, emphasis added)

Other reports, published the same year, however, identified the experimental nature of cochlear implantation:

> The 24-year-old Studio City man is one of a few hundred people worldwide to take part in the experimental use of a hearing aid that is implanted in his head. . . . "I never got my hopes up really high," said Meier, who was warned by doctors that the device might help him only slightly or not at all. (Wharton 1986, 24)

* * *

> The new 22-channel model Cochlear Nucleus 22 can carry a wider range of frequencies and volume levels than earlier implants, but it's still experimental and will require fine-tuning, Kileny said. (*Chicago Tribune* 1986, 3)

By 1987, the program was still clearly at an experimental stage (Cameron and Steinhauer 1987, 1), and profoundly deaf U.S. veterans were sought to participate in a $3 million study to evaluate the effectiveness of four different types of cochlear implants, provided free to participants in the study (Kotulak and Van 1987). The benefits were claimed to be that some patients were "now able to listen to their grandchildren singing. They now hear airplanes and sometimes even birds" (*The Baton Rouge Sunday Advocate* 1989). Other than one article that described implantation simplistically as having "given hearing back to twenty-seven patients" (Thomas 1987, 4), reports became more qualified in the sensational benefits of implantation and more specific in their reporting of the actual results experienced by recipients.

> They help people hear environmental sounds such as sirens and doorbells, but don't supply clear renditions of conversations. (Van 1987, 15)
>
> * * *
>
> Cochlear implants for the profoundly deaf, though the "artificial ear" is anything but a miracle cure [sic]. The electronic device, implanted within the ear, alerts the wearer to noise—say, an approaching car. Some training is necessary to learn to use the sounds intelligently. (Walker 1987, 16)
>
> * * *
>
> "Compared to [sic] a normal ear, these are very rudimentary devices," Dr. McCabe said. (*U.S.A. Today* 1987)

That same year, an article described the difficulty the University of California (UC) cochlear implantation program had experienced in the 1970s with malfunctions in its experimental implanted equipment, a problem it claimed was now solved (Petit 1987, 24). UC San Francisco planned to begin clinical trials of its new eight-channel implant the following year (Times Wire Services 1987); however, cochlear implantation programs generally were still experiencing difficulty attracting candidates:

> Despite evidence that the devices help and that they are steadily improving, many deaf people who are good candidates for the procedure turn it down. "We were literally unable to get any cochlear implant subjects to work with," said Dr. Blair Simmons, a hearing specialist and surgeon at Stanford University Medical Center, where he conducted cochlear implant research before giving it up recently. Distinct improvement in cochlear implant performance is seen as vital if more patients are to agree to have them implanted. The procedure requires from two to six hours of surgery and costs $20,000 or more for both the device and medical expenses. (Petit 1987, 24)

Although the outcomes of adult implantation were still largely unknown or unpredictable, in 1987, the FDA approved its use in adults, resulting in reportedly 600 adults receiving cochlear implants worldwide (*The Omaha World-Herald* 1987). The doctors continued to express uncertainty in the outcomes that could be expected:

When they had their surgeries, the men knew there were no guarantees they would be able to hear anything after the instrumentation was activated. "One lady wanted to mortgage her house, and I told her no because if the operation doesn't work you will have no hearing and no house," Toso said. "First, we don't know if it will work because we don't know how many electrodes will work. One of our patients with the multi-channel implant only has one electrode working. You have to be certain you have a clear understanding. We hope to be able to get some result, but we cannot guarantee how much. Each patient has a different response." . . . [S]urgeons don't really know what will be possible until they see the patient's cochlea. (Griffiths 1989, 1)

The same year that the FDA approved adult implantation (1987), childhood implantation was being permitted on an experimental basis (Baker 1988), and there were about twenty children worldwide who had received a cochlear implant (*The Omaha World-Herald* 1987). The experimental nature of childhood implantation was widely reported, with claims of the following anticipated benefits:

Jayson is one of a handful of children around the world to get an experimental device called a "cochlear implant" which some doctors believe has the potential to bring hearing to thousands of deaf people. (Brody 1988, 1)

Doctors were unsure of what outcomes to expect for children who had been deaf since birth. Commenting on two such children, U.S. doctors (cited in *The Omaha World-Herald* 1987) reportedly said:

"They can hear sound. We don't know if they are going to be able to make these sounds into speech" [and] "We'll have to wait and see. . . . We're not worried about quantity right now. . . . We are in the research mode." (n.p.)

Other doctors expressed outcomes cautiously:

"We don't tell parents their children will be able to talk, but some are developing speech and language." (Saltus 1989, 27)

* * *

"We didn't know whether this whole thing was going to be a real fizzer. [The outcome with] Pia could have been absolutely awful and a total failure," he [Professor Bill Gibson, cochlear implant surgeon at Children's Hospital, Sydney] said. "But it has been a success and shows we have progressed from the experimental to clinical phase with children." (Prior 1988, 2)

* * *

There is much debate about the effectiveness of cochlear implants in children. Experimental studies are under way at several institutions around the country to determine the device's worth in children of all ages who have profound hearing loss. Conner [Dr. George Conner, chief of otolaryngology at Hershey Medical Center, central Pennsylvania] said it is not yet known if congenitally deaf children with implants will be signers or learn to speak. (Griffiths 1989, 1)

Parents' expectations ranged from the romantic to pragmatic—expecting their child to hear music, hoping the child would gain enough hearing to be warned of an approaching vehicle, and anticipating an improved chance of higher education.

> "Now he'll hear all the beautiful sounds . . . the music," the father says. "And if the birds chirp loud enough, he'll hear them too." (Mills 1985)

> * * *

> All Mrs. Ingalls dares hope is that someday her son would be able to hear something approaching, such as a speeding car or a fire engine, thus saving his life. (Brody 1988, 5)

> * * *

> He may never be mainstreamed into the public school system and his speech will probably always sound different. But one day the Sunderlands hope their son will go to college. (Karkabi 1988)

> * * *

> "Nikki had to have it for her education and well-being," Mrs. Savage said. "If nothing else, to see the look on her face when she hears herself screaming" (Tuck 1989a, 2)

Reported Outcomes of Implantation

The reported outcomes of implantation in the daily press generally fall into two categories: anecdotal and science-based. The first category is largely personal interest stories, at times sensationalized (or simplistic), often emotive, and reported without reference to scientific study. The second group of articles reports the findings of scientific research that generally has been funded and undertaken by implant developers. Making a distinction between the cochlear implant industry and cochlear implant scientific community is often difficult.

Anecdotal Reports

Anecdotal reports of the outcomes of cochlear implantation have been all too common in the daily press in most nations. Personal interest stories and the use of emotive language, abound.

The word *miracle* is closely associated with press reports of the outcomes of implantation. More often than not, these reports are the interpretation of reporters or the creation of byline editors who attract readers' attention through sensational headlines:

- "Man given ear implant able to detect sound after 50 years silence" (Immen 1984)
- "Experimental implant rescues man from years of deafness" (Feldman 1985, 5)
- "Many deaf prefer static to silence, but others expected to hear Beethoven" (Mills 1985)

- "Every noise is a pleasure to once-deaf man" (United Press International 1985) (In this article, the implant recipient, Clark Berke, reportedly "flushes the toilet repeatedly, slams doors, crinkles paper, taps his fingers on wood and smiles frequently.")
- "College student's hearing restored by surgically implanted hearing device" (*The Seattle Times* 1985)
- "New implant opens world of sound for deaf people" (Associated Press 1985, 3)
- "Nikki, 6, recovering from first step toward regaining her hearing" (Tuck 1989b, J2) and, six weeks later, "Little Nikki's world is silent no more: 6-year-old's hearing restored with surgery" (Tuck 1989a, J2)

Some parents and even professionals working in the cochlear implant industry also represent implantation as a "miracle" or "gift of God." For example, after her husband received a cochlear implant, the wife of an American judge described it as an "absolute miracle" (Dreyfuss 1985, 1).[1] And the parents of two U.S. children at a press conference for cochlear implantation said, "We are thrilled to death . . . We thank the Lord that He's given Tim some ears" and "Toni couldn't hear at all. . . . She's quite aware now that there is sound in the air. Whether she ever talks or not is not the point" (*The Omaha World-Herald* 1987, n.p.). The clinical director of auditory therapy at North York General Hospital, Warren Estabrooks, described implantation in similar terms: a "modern-day miracle" and "like a scene from the miracle worker" (Murray 1989, 11).

A dominant approach used in reports on cochlear implantation has been to use emotive language and to describe those sounds ostensibly most cherished by hearing people (music, bird song, and so on) and previously unavailable to deaf or hearing impaired people. The outcome of implantation is often described in terms of communication in a limited number of domains—principally, the use of language to express feelings. The reader is left with the impression that deafness negates the ability to communicate such emotion through other means (such as gesture and signed language), thus heightening the reader's emotional response to the benefits of implantation. The following example, from the first of many articles about this implant recipient, comes from the Australian press:

> Pia Jeffrey can hear for the first time—and it's written all over her face. Now she knows the voices of her mother, father and sister. "Pia, Pia, I love you," her mother said. . . . Her speech level is still about that of a two-year-old. Professor Gibson said he hopes that one day she will master the use of language. But she has already heard the most important words. "Pia, I love you." (Cameron and Steinhauer 1987, 1)

Another example comes from the *St. Petersburg Times*. The child in this article is described as a "blond, dimpled charmer" who cried when he was deaf and, after implantation, signed "I can hear, I can hear!"

> The blond, dimpled charmer understood from an early age that his parents could listen to his cries, that somehow he was missing something. "I want to hear," he motioned to them in sign language as soon as he knew how . . .

---

1. The article received vigorous response from Deaf people (see Miller 1985 and Porco 1985).

"We'd prepared ourselves for the worst," Mrs. Ingalls recalls. "We expected him to cry and try to throw the cord away in fear. But he kept signing to us, "I can hear, I can hear." When we got home, he jumped out of the car to show his friends. . . . At school he's doing fine, too. When Jayson first responded to her call, his teacher, Kathleen Loftus, remembers it as the most rewarding day of her career. "I hugged him to death," said Loftus, who teaches Jayson's class of eight hearing-impaired . . . "and still cry every time I think about it." (Brody 1988, 5)

* * *

She knows she'll never be able to hear the full range of sound of a wood thrush, much less the complex sound pattern of a symphony orchestra. . . . It sends her its version of all sounds—say a cricket's chirping (Signor 1989, D1).

Within the category of anecdotal reports of the outcomes of cochlear implantation, the final group of reports comprises those that include no reference to scientific study. Bald statements appear in the press that either make claims for cochlear implantation without reference to research evidence or use language that has a high degree of uncertainty.

For six-year-old Nikki Savage, a Winder girl who recently underwent implant surgery to have her hearing restored, the hardest part was the haircut. (Tuck 1989b, J2)

* * *

So far, he can't recognize many words besides his name, but he's starting to count by listening to drum beats. He can't pronounce many words, either, but is beginning to imitate speech sounds. (Brody 1988, 1 5)

* * *

"He's very intelligent and has a great willingness to learn," Loftus [who teaches Jayson's class of eight hard of hearing students at Tampa's Cahoon Elementary School] said. "As long as he's into it and wants to talk and hear, he will." (Brody 1988, 1, 5)

* * *

There are no guarantees, but implants have helped restore partial hearing to thousands of adults and 170 children nationwide. (Tuck 1989b, J2)

* * *

I would have hoped the sounds I would get from it would be more normal sounds than that [sic] actually are," [said Robert Buxton, an adult cochlear implant recipient]. (Griffiths 1989, 1)

More commonly, the outcomes of implantation have been reported as the "return of hearing," examples of which refer only to the recognition of environmental sounds:

- the ring of the telephone, the dial tone, and her own voice (Rabkin 1982, 13)
- dogs barking, crickets singing, birds chirping, the wind, the water sprinkler (Feldman 1985, 5)
- cars, trains, footsteps, sirens, and telephones (Johnson 1985, 7)

- birds singing, her own footsteps, car horns honking, telephones ringing, or doors closing (O'Neill 1985, 18)
- street sounds, a baby cry, or simple words like yes and no (Thompson 1985, 12)
- birds singing, the wind, the rain, kids laughing, a passing skateboard, sirens, cars honking, a helicopter flying overhead (Wharton 1986, 24)
- the difference between sound and silence (Karkabi 1988)
- a door slamming, the phone ringing, speech (without the support of speech-reading) (Pollack 1988, D1)
- the doorbell, the phone, the difference between the pump for the well and the furnace that heats the house, the click of the car's turn signal when stopped at a red light or stop sign (Griffiths 1989, 1)
- birds singing, cars, and plates clinking (Lumby 1989, 17)
- the sound of a kettle boiling (Murray 1989, 11)
- traffic going by on the street, the school bell, a teacher calling for attention, the bustling and closing of books when a class is over, water running in the sink, the clock chiming on the hour (Signor 1989, D1)

The sounds themselves have been described by implant recipients or their doctors as

- "buzzes and hums" (Immen 1984, M7),
- "a crude buzzing in his forehead" (Mills 1985, n.p.),
- "muffled" (Signor 1989, D1),
- "buzzes or beeps" (O'Neill 1985, 18),
- a "scratchy clicking noise similar to static interference on a radio that is not quite tuned in" (Thompson 1985, 12),
- sounding like "a radio not quite tuned in" (Ricks 1986, 1),
- "kind of fuzzy . . . like listening to an AM radio from ten feet away" (Wharton 1986, 24),
- sounding "like Donald Duck talking under water (Cameron and Steinhauer 1987, 1),
- "a monotone sound, like a bee's buzzing" (Scripps 1988, 1),
- sounding "like hearing voices underwater" (Karkabi 1988),
- sounding "like listening to a static-ridden radio," (a phrase like "How are you?" likely to come across as "ba ba boo") (Randal 1988b, 11), and
- a "whirl of nonsense sounds in his head" (referring to music; Griffiths 1989, 1).

Overall, the results were largely unknown:

We call it an artificial ear, but it isn't. We think of it as a miracle that can allow the deaf to hear, but it can't. It does something else. Public television's look at the cochlear implant . . . underscores the limitations of medical technology while celebrating the promise. Dale's [an adult implant recipient] early frustrations are contrasted to [sic] the remarkable success of an Austrian woman who has worn a similar implant for four years. With a Mozart horn concerto providing the background music, Sonja [the Austrian woman] is shown taking part in normal conversations and doing well in a hearing test.

"Sonja is lucky," narrator Peter Graves says, "a real star in the world of cochlear implant patients." Her implant, made by 3M, uses a different speech-processing computer than [sic] Dale's, although that does not explain her success. The technology is too new for doctors to be able to predict when an implant will succeed and when it will fail. (Berg 1985a, 20)

Science-Based Reports

The second category of articles identified in this analysis comprises reports from the cochlear implant industry and from the cochlear implant scientific community. An article published by *The Boston Globe* (Saltus 1989, 27) claimed that researchers reported anecdotal results, often emphasizing successes, and that careful scientific studies were not yet complete. Some reports were vague enough to make them of little use, or they used language with a low level of modality such as "a significant number," "can," "varying amounts of," "some," and "significant success," as in the following examples (emphasis added):

- [Tests on about 2,000 deaf patients showed] *"a significant number* of them are now able to recognize speech." (Lufkin 1988, 3)
- [The multichannel (Nucleus 22) device] *"can* restore sound and speech recognition to profoundly deaf people." (*Business Wire* 1989)
- "Only fourteen children in the country [the United States] have had the procedure with *varying amounts* of improvement." (Bown 1989, 06)
- [Cochlear implants] can restore sound and speech recognition in *some* profoundly deaf individuals. (Griffiths 1989, 1)
- Cochlear implant surgery . . . literally brings back the "sounds of life" to persons who have been totally deaf. Recent significant success has been achieved with children. (*Canada News-Wire* 1989)

The results reported by the cochlear implant developers and manufacturers generally fall into two broad groups: (a) reports claiming that its device made deaf people aware of environmental sounds and, in conjunction with training and speechreading, could allow deaf people to understand speech more clearly—generally representing the results of single-channel devices (see Mills 1984; Perlman 1985, 3), the results achieved by postlingual deaf adults, or both (Gindick 1985, 1)—and (b) reports claiming that the device enabled speech awareness, with and without the help of speechreading. The following conclusions were drawn by U.S. federal experts at a National Institutes of Health meeting, showing an example of the first broad group:

The implants do not cure profound deafness, but they do improve the perception of sound, alerting users to environmental noises: a doorbell, a dog's bark or an auto horn. They also make lip-reading easier, and in about 5 percent of cases users can converse with a nearby person whose back is turned. Some of these hearing-impaired people can even use the telephone with relative ease. (Randal 1988b, 11)

Additional examples representing the first group reflect views of other co-chlear implant professionals who issued warnings and called for caution:

[The cochlear implant] enables people once totally deaf to hear voices but is not discriminating enough to permit understanding of words that are spoken. (Molotsky 1984, 1)

* * *

A Chicago otologist . . . won't yet recommend cochlear implants. "We're all hoping something will come of this," Dr. Harrison says. But not until the de-vices can discriminate speech "could I tell my patients in all honesty that it could work for them." (Mills 1985, n.p.)

* * *

The newly developed cochlear implant receives sound signals and translates them into electrical impulses to be sent to the auditory nerve, which carries signals to the brain. . . . "Patients with implanted nerve stimulators should be warned of the possibility of . . . interference," Hepfner [Sharon Hepfner of the University of Cincinnati Medical Center] writes, "and should be alert to the presence of radio transmitters, library and airport metal detectors, and electrical sources capable of emitting appreciable radio-frequency energy." Most important, she writes, these people need to be assured that they are not imagining the sounds. (Berg 1985b, 05)

* * *

"At best, the device allows only a rough approximation of normal hearing," he [Jeff Burres, executive director of the Davenport Medical Center] said. Therefore, recipients cannot fully understand such sounds as music or speech over a telephone, nor can they follow a conversation without lip-reading. (*The Omaha World-Herald* 1986, n.p.)

* * *

Responding to a question put to him in his medical column for the *Chicago Tribune*, a doctor advised patients to lower their expectations: "Some patients expect too much from the implant and are disappointed with the results. Deaf patients who obtain the hearing device cannot expect to hear as well as they once did naturally. Sounds are often muffled or seem to contain static. But for many who get the implant, even the slightest bit of noise sounds beauti-ful." (Bruckheim 1987, 8)

* * *

Director of a research institute at the University of Michigan, Dr. Josef M. Miller, reported that some implant recipients may be able to understand a simple request over the telephone but "they can't have a conversation of the kind we're having now." (Special Correspondent 1987, n.p.)

* * *

In 1988, a time at which childhood implantation was being conducted on an experimental basis, doctors reported that implantation posed "a slight risk of infection and facial paralysis." (Brody 1988, 1)

* * *

Only about 5 percent of implant recipients could carry on a normal conversation without speech reading. . . . Some people are improved just a little, others spectacularly, and we do not know why there is that difference. . . . Some people can detect only sounds like a door slamming or the phone ringing. Others can do as well as to understand speech without lip-reading and talking on the phone. (Pollack 1988, D1)

* * *

"There is a real danger of overselling implants," said Richard S. Stoker, Director of the Central Institute for the Deaf in St. Louis. He is concerned that hospitals will undertake implant programs as a "profit-oriented thing" without recognizing the need for extensive—and costly—counseling and rehabilitation for implant patients. (Saltus 1989, 27)

* * *

"Most of the candidates do have unrealistic expectations. They hope to hear perfectly, and yes, they are saddened when this isn't the case. The person has to be aware of possibly only attaining a small degree of benefit. They have to be prepared for any degree of outcome." (Elca Swigart, clinical audiologist and director of the Speech and Hearing Center, Reading Hospital and Medical Center, Pennsylvania, quoted in, cited in Griffiths 1989, 1)

* * *

I would have hoped the sounds I would get from [the implant] would be more normal sounds than they actually are. (Adult implant recipient quoted in Griffiths 1989, 1)

* * *

"Deaf individuals must mourn the loss of their hearing and come to terms with it before being considered as implantation candidates," Mills [coordinator of the Adult Cochlear Implant Patient Division, Los Angeles Otologic Medical Group] said. "The person who has not adjusted to existing in a world of silence could have great difficulty accepting another disappointment should he or she be among the 1 percent of implant patients who receive no auditory information from the device," she said. (Griffiths 1989, 1)

* * *

By the late 1980s, the outcomes of cochlear implantation were still generally unknown. The U.S. federal panel of experts who met at a National Institutes of Health meeting (mentioned above) concluded the following:

"Cochlear prostheses are good and are going to get better," said the panel's chairman, Dr. Robert I. Kohut, a professor of otolaryngology at the Bowman Gray School of Medicine, Winston-Salem, N.C. The technology still has some distance to go. For one thing, it is now impossible to tell in advance how much an implant will help an individual. As one panel member put it, "Some implant users are stars, but others derive little benefit from the devices, and still others find them so annoying that they turn them off." (Randal 1988b, 11)

And Saltus (1989, 27) reported: "Cochlear implants, the closest thing yet to an artificial ear, are coming into their own after years of experiment and controversy. Compared with natural hearing, the implants provide crude and sometimes meaningless sound, and results vary enormously in different patients."

The second group of results reported by developers and manufacturers is that the device enabled speech awareness, with and without the help of speechreading:

- The Ineraid implant had been tested on one profoundly deaf person, and the company reported that, after several years, he was able to hear and understand 80 percent of two-syllable words without the help of speechreading and 90 percent to 100 percent with speechreading (Chase 1984b).
- The following conclusion from a study published in the journal *Medical Progress through Technology* was reported in the daily press: "It is possible to reestablish some understanding of open speech through the use of the cochlear implant without additional lipreading" (Berg 1985a, 20).
- An audiologist at Symbion, Dr. Korine Dankowski, reported that eleven of the implant recipients tested scored an average of 97 percent on everyday sentence tests using both auditory and visual clues, an average of 26 percent on similar studies without speechreading; six of the eleven, deaf for fifteen years or less, averaged 41 percent without speechreading (PR Newswire 1985b).
- Tests with a multifrequency model had shown that "some completely deaf people can hear and recognize up to 75 percent of words spoken to them without any visual cues" (Thompson 1985, 12).
- Two Sydney hospitals (the Royal Prince Alfred Hospital and St Vincent's Hospital) reported that their device enabled 15 percent of recipients to use a telephone adequately, another 50 percent to carry on a conversation, and the remaining 35 percent to understand by using a combination of the implant and speechreading (Thomas 1986, 3).
- Clinical director of the University of California San Francisco cochlear implant project, Dr. Robert Schindler, reported that all but three of his sixteen patients implanted with a four-channel device could understand some speech: "Seven of the patients scored 50 percent or better on standard tests of speech recognition without lip reading. . . . These high percentages of speech recognition appear to be unique among the various cochlear implant research groups. . . . These patients can clearly distinguish human speech, rather than just hearing sound, as is the case with some implants" (Times Wire Services 1987, 21).
- Otolaryngologist and co-developer of the Clarion cochlear implant, Dr. Robert Schindler, reported that the implant had been fitted in eighteen patients and was very successful:

> In clinical tests, seven of these patients understood half the common words and sentences without lip-reading. Eight could understand at least a quarter of monosyllabic words. All improved their lip-reading ability. When compared with others at an international symposium in West Germany last September, these were "the best results in the world," Schindler said. "Maybe two or three out of hundreds of other implants perform at that level," he said. Schindler said that experiments with this particular design were not continuing because "we know how to make it better." This year,

clinical trials begin on an eight-channel design able to transmit more frequencies. The best candidates for the cochlear implant now, Schindler said, are totally deaf adults who can't benefit from hearing aids. He looks forward to the possibility of extending it to children and the congenitally deaf. Bringing sounds and words back to people and watching their reaction is "one of the most moving things I've ever seen," he said. (Stuart 1988, 7)

By the late 1980s, there were reportedly 500 people throughout the world who had been implanted (Slee 1987).

THE SHIFTING CRITERIA FOR IMPLANTATION

Single-channel implants were approved by the FDA for clinical use in adults in 1985. Reports at the time clearly indicated that cochlear implantation was intended to assist "those with profound hearing loss who could not benefit from conventional hearing aids" (Johnson 1985, 7). The focus was on individuals who had developed normal speech but had acquired a profound hearing loss. It was reported that cochlear implants could "only be used in patients who have had some hearing during their lives" (Thomas 1986, 3) and that "those who have congenital deafness or who never developed normal speech before developing profound hearing loss probably would not benefit from cochlear implant surgery" (Johnson 1985, 7). For implantation to go ahead, adults needed to meet the following criteria: have profound hearing loss in both ears, receive no benefit from hearing aids, have acquired spoken language before their hearing loss, have no other serious medical conditions, have the support of families and friends, and have a "true desire to become part of the hearing community" (Griffiths 1989, 1). The following year, the FDA approved the experimental use of cochlear implants with ten- to seventeen-year-olds and the experimental use of the twenty-two-channel device (Wharton 1986, 24).

The first shift in criteria from the implantation of profoundly deaf adults with acquired hearing loss came in 1987. In that year, the first U.S. citizen, deaf from infancy, received a cochlear implant (*U.S.A. Today* 1987), and the FDA granted approval for Cochlear Corporation to implant up to seventy-five hearing impaired people (Galarneau 1988, 3). An indication of the industry's interest in (and the inevitability of) childhood implantation had been flagged in the mid-1980s and was clearly on the agenda by the late 1980s. For example, as early as 1985, one commentator predicted: "As we gain more experience with people who have normal speech and language, there is no question that this device will have enormous impact on deaf children" (Associated Press 1985, 3). In 1987, another article reported: "I think the implant is probably one of the best suited (operations) for profoundly deaf children," he [Dr. Herman Jenkins, an ear, nose, and throat specialist at Baylor College of Medicine, Houston] said. "If you get sound to them at an early age, there is a much better chance of learning language" (Millsap 1987, 16).

Experimental implantation of children was ongoing through the late 1980s (Griffiths 1989), and though not yet approved for wider use, the expectation was that it would be within one to two years. U.S. otologist Dr. Charles Mangham, was reported to say: "It will be approved [by the FDA]; it's just a matter of when" (*The Seattle Times* 1988, 4; see also Roan 1989).

Australian researchers had already indicated their plans to do implantation in children younger than the age of three (Slee 1987). In 1988, a Sydney University researcher, Dr. Gaye Nicholls, announced an "exciting breakthrough"; after studying (just) four children who had received an Australian implant, she reported that cochlear implants "would enable many profoundly deaf children to hear and learn to speak instead of relying on sign language and lip-reading" (*Sydney Morning Herald* 1988, 8). However, this expectation of success was not shared by all Australian researchers:

> There's another group, those born deaf, who have never heard anything at all, never developed the ability to understand speech using hearing. It's questionable whether doing surgery and putting this complicated device into their head is worth while," says [Professor] Dowell. "Because they've never had sound before it seems unlikely that later in life they'd be able to learn to understand hearing." (Brown 1989, n.p.)

There was support for childhood implantation in the United States. For example, Ralph Naunton, director of research at the National Institute of Deafness and Other Communication Disorders in Bethesda, Maryland, indicated support for childhood implantation, saying that it took advantage of "a valuable time window when you can teach them speech and get language into them" (Saltus 1989, 27), although he acknowledged that it was "still too soon to draw conclusions about implants' effectiveness in children lacking language abilities" (27). Researchers were hoping the implants "may allow them to develop some degree of oral language" (27) to children who were born deaf.

The requirements for childhood implantation began with parents, the school, audiologists, and physicians "needing to agree after extensive testing that a child will probably benefit from the surgery" (Millsap 1987, 16). Other experts were reported as saying, "An implant should be considered . . . only if the child first fails to benefit from at least six months of auditory training with a conventional hearing aid" (Randal 1988b, 11). Randal's article went on to say:

> If it is then decided to go ahead, the decision should be based on thorough medical and psychological evaluation and an understanding that the child will have to refrain from contact sports and will still need special education and other support services for the hearing-impaired. (1988b, 11)

According to Randal, more than 3,000 cochlear implants had been implanted in patients around the world, most of whom were American adults (Randal 1988b).

TECHNOLOGICAL DEVELOPMENTS

The acknowledged gap between the potential of current technology and results from studies of recipients implanted with a previous-generation device continues to be problematic. The pace of technology is rapid and has generally advanced faster than research results can be made available. Although critics of cochlear implants raised questions about the outcomes of cochlear implantation, the response they got was often that the study in question related to older generation devices and that current technology was much more advanced. For some years, before the multichannel implant became the industry standard, there was fierce competition among implant producers and clear benefits for those who were implanted with more sophisticated devices. It seems reasonable that the Deaf community and others cautious of implantation would question where this rapidly changing technology left the many recipients who had been part of the experimental or early implant programs in which they had received (what were later regarded as) "inferior" devices. This kind of rapid change was one of the reasons given for the reluctance of some specialists to implant children:

> So far, the cochlear implant isn't for kids. . . . Although some implants have been functioning for six years, there is no telling how long they'll go on working. Doctors prefer not to have children undergo the implantation because they may eventually require several operations. Additionally, better devices may be available soon. (O'Neill 1985, 18)

By 1985, there were reportedly 665 people, including 164 children, who had been implanted with the single-channel 3M House implant (Dreyfuss 1985). Several articles, represented in the following quotes, were published at this time, reporting the inferiority of this model.

> Single-channel implants are "better than nothing, but that's all they are— better than nothing," said Daniel Ling, who is serving as a consultant to an Australian company, Nucleus Group, developing a 22-channel cochlear implant device. . . . "Why implant a single-channel today if you know a 22-channel is right around the corner?" (Mills 1984)

* * *

> Until now, a one-channel version has been used, translating sounds into clicks and buzzes. The four-channel device is like "the difference between hitting all the keys of the piano at once or playing one key at a time," says Dr. Robert Schindler of the University of California at San Francisco. (Berg 1985c, 5)

* * *

> Tests of an improved [four-channel] electronic implant that can simulate hearing have begun in California, and researchers are hopeful that it will allow some deaf people to understand speech. (Berg 1985c, 5)

* * *

> "Single channel implants were the first, but they made people aware mainly only of noise, because there was only one tone that you could turn on and off," [Dr.] Davidson said. (Smollar 1986, 5)

* * *

> One-channel implants gave patients sound awareness. The multichannel implant extracts features of speech that resemble fairly normal sound. (Millsap 1987, 16)

* * *

"The new [eight-channel] device may give deaf patients improved ability to recognize speech and may broaden the opportunity for success in patients who received only minimal benefit from the four-channel implant," Schindler said. "If an implant provides only single channel stimulation, the patient may hear some environmental and a few speech sounds, but complete speech recognition is highly unlikely." (Times Wire Services 1987, 21)

* * *

"Most of the implants that are in use now are the single-channel variety that, while useful, didn't give people speech as such—they gave them sound awareness and better lip-reading," Pulec said. "The multichannel units truly offer to the average patient a reasonable improvement. They get somewhere between 30 percent and 70 percent understanding of words." (Baker 1988, 4)

It had been reported that "about 30 percent of the adults born deaf who tried implants quit using them after a short time" (Dreyfuss 1985, 1). Unlike the views of the above researchers, Dr. William House, the inventor of the 3M House implant, used different reasons to explain the unpopularity of his device among people born deaf:

"People born deaf feel safer in their own environment," House said. "They have never known the hearing environment. To many born deaf, the hearing world is threatening and alien. It ignores the deaf and often is annoyed by them. There is a defensive sense of alienation and, sometimes, superiority among some born deaf. They have their lives, their culture, which is not understood by the hearing," House said. (Dreyfuss 1985, 1)

Another issue of contention between cochlear implant advocates and those opposed to or wary of implantation is the targeted media selection of implant recipients with the express purpose to promote cochlear implantation. The following media reports promote the strategic selections of those who perform well with an implant and the overwhelming silence over those who do not perform well or have adverse affects from an implant:

Dr. Warren Brandes, an Ear, Nose and Throat specialist who gave Berke the implant, said . . . he chose Berke for the operation because Berke is smart and motivated and has a lot of support from his family. (United Press International 1985)

* * *

"I think the good Lord smiled on us when he sent us John," he [Dr. J. Stephen Sinclair, an associate professor at California State Univesity, Northridge] said. "He's extremely intelligent and highly motivated. He has a supportive family. He's the ideal patient." (Wharton 1986, 24)

FINANCIAL IMPERATIVES

"Our no. 1 revenue priority," Dr. Jarvik says, "is getting the artificial ear to market." (Chase 1984a)

Financial support for the development of the cochlear implant industry came from several quarters. To develop their business, implant manufacturers required access to millions of dollars in research and development funds, approval from federal agencies such as the FDA, and ways for potential customers to access financial support (through government-funded or privately funded medical schemes). In many cases, the families of young children accessed funds through public or private appeals.

The *Business Atlanta* reported: "You can do almost anything if you have unlimited funds, or if it's worth it in the payback. It's a matter of looking at economic feasibility of new product innovations and deciding how fast you can move based on that economic feasibility" (Shaw 1985, 98). Canada's implant program was reportedly supported by the Medical Research Council of Canada, the Physicians Services Incorporated, the Natural Sciences and Engineering Research Council, and the Masonic Foundation of Ontario (Immen 1984).

In 1984, Australian high-technology group Nucleus sent a representative, Mike Hirshorn, to the United States to open up a market for the company's cochlear implant. *Business Review Weekly* reported: "Hirshorn had to contend with some formidable obstacles, including a tough regulatory authority, the U.S. Food and Drug Administration, and a determined market leader, 3M" (Kavanagh 1988, 62). Within four years, the company built an 80 percent share of the U.S. market and, in 1988, built a 35 percent share of the European market (Kavanagh 1988). To challenge the dominance of 3M, which marketed the single-channel implant, Hirshorn approached leading clinical surgeons to implant his company's device on a trial basis, promising technical support within the United States within one day. He also "pursued high-level contacts in U.S. medical associations and professional groups to help smooth the way to FDA approval" (Kavanagh 1988, 62).

After receiving FDA approval for the implantation of adults in 1985, another crucial breakthrough for the industry was gaining approval from national medical schemes and private health insurers. The U.S. Medicare scheme approved refunds up to $8,000 for cochlear implantation in 1986 (Wharton 1986); the Australian Medicare scheme provided adult implantation free of charge from 1987 (Thomas 1987). Before gaining this approval, a rash of articles appeared in the press, pushing for universal medical coverage for cochlear implant patients. Most made the point expressed in the following example:

> Medicare is allegedly a universal health scheme but these patients, who cannot afford the costs of the device or insurance, are just left to sit and wait while patients with the required money are able to get the implants and hear again. (Thomas 1986, 3)

U.S. and Australian cochlear implant companies faced a critical period in 1987. Despite a heavily advertised program in the United States to attract patients with hearing disorders, American insurance companies had been slow to add cochlear implantation to their approved coverage. The same year, the FDA recalled the implant, removing about 8 percent of the hospitals' $12 million annual budget (Schroer 1987). That year, experimental procedures were paid for by insurance, Medicare, and part of a $2.6 million federal grant (*The Omaha World-Herald* 1987). The following year, sales were still below expectations; one reason attributed to the limited market success was that "the outcome of the implant is unpredictable"

(*HealthWeek* 1988, 19). The implant and associated medical costs were estimated at upward of $25,000 (Pollack 1988), and some health insurance programs were holding out:

> "We're just not convinced yet that it still isn't experimental surgery," said Dr. Glen Taylor, a consultant in the benefits branch of Medi-Cal, California's health insurance program for the indigent. "The evidence for good is still outweighed by the bad." (Baker 1988, 4)
>
> * * *
>
> A 3-year-old . . . boy is scheduled for surgery Wednesday to receive an experimental device that may restore his speech and hearing, but his family faces a struggle after an insurance company refused to cover the operation's costs. . . . [T]he estimated $22,000 cost of the surgery and follow-up treatment likely will be borne by his parents, because his insurance company won't pay for experimental devices. . . . The health-maintenance organization denied coverage because the device has not received final food and drug administration approval for use in children. "Our position is that the way our contracts are written throughout the country . . . experimental or investigational devices are not covered," said Dave Anderson, director of operations for Foundation Health's Spokane Division. (*The Seattle Times* 1988, B4).

In Melbourne, the acting chairman of the Australian Bionic Ear Institute, Dr. Field Rickards, was reported to say that "lack of funds and laboratories could prevent Australia from staying in the forefront of bionic ear development." The institute sought $2 million corporate sponsorship to set up seven new laboratories to continue its research or "the rest of the world was likely to catch up with developments [in Victoria]" (Slee 1987, 13). Two years later, Cochlear Corporation, with the world's leading share of the cochlear implant market, purchased 3M, the U.S. manufacturer of House implants (*Business Wire* 1989).

Some parents of potential recipients were willing to put themselves into debt to fund their child's implantation; others sought charitable donations.

> "Our insurance will not cover this," said Debbie Savage, Nikki's mother. "If it cost $2 million dollars I would pay the rest of my life and sell everything." (Bown 1989)
>
> * * *
>
> "We're putting our life savings down and making payments," said his father. (*The Seattle Times* 1988, 4)
>
> * * *
>
> His fund-raising efforts to help 5-year-old Ryan Odland, deaf since birth, get a much-needed ear operation, go well beyond sympathy. Clemens, owner and operator of Clemens Laboratories, a baby products manufacturing company, has taken it upon himself to raise the money needed for the $25,000 operation. (Pemberton-Reid 1987)
>
> * * *
>
> "There were so many times I felt like throwing in the towel," said Mrs. Ingalls, recalling 15 hours a week of begging for donations from any organi-

zation that came to mind. Then I'd look at Jayson and think, "How am I going to tell him he can't hear because nobody wants to pay?" The crucial boost came this spring when she called Farrukh Quraishi, who used to play soccer with the Tampa Bay Rowdies. He arranged for the team to play in a benefit game in March that raised more than $2,000. Friends at MacDill pitched in as well, and when the doctors decided to donate their services, cutting the $25,000 bill in half, they had enough money to proceed. (Brody 1988, 5)

* * *

Cap off the St. George Lantern Club's Celebrity Golf Day, which will raise more than $30,000 for the Royal NSW [New South Wales] Institute for Deaf and Blind Children at North Rocks. In particular, the money will go to the Sydney University Cochlear Implant . . . Program. (*Sun Herald* 1988, 96)

* * *

Celebrities from a television station in Atlanta will challenge Gwinnett Medical Center in a benefit slow-pitch softball game Saturday to help pay a local girl's medical expenses. (Bown 1989, J6)

* * *

Pledges will be donated to the Rotary Hearing Centre which supports research and funding to restore hearing for persons who are totally deaf. (*Canada News-Wire* 1989)

* * *

Since the implant surgery is not covered by the family's insurance, friends and co-workers of Mrs. Savage at Gwinnett Medical Center in Lawrenceville have raised about $18,000. Fund-raisers still are being held for the family, said Mrs. Savage. Despite the financial impact of the surgery, the Savages have no regrets about their decision to have Nikki undergo implant surgery. (Tuck 1989a, J2)

* * *

The high school raised $4,000 towards the implant and the musical director wrote a musical about deafness for Sam which the school performed when he arrived back from hospital. (Lumby 1989, 17)

* * *

At $100 a head and with 2,000 capacity in what is expected to be a sellout . . . they are hoping to raise $200,000 for the St. Louis Children's Hospital's Cochlear Implant Program. (Dames 1989, S4)

The FDA approved implantation in children in 1990. The cochlear implant industry, through a number of measures, including the promotion of cochlear implantation through the press, has succeeded in promoting childhood implantation. A key approach was to use success stories or, as they are sometimes called, their "stars":

"A lot of patients don't really know that the device is available," said Judith Brimacombe, a clinical coordinator for Cochlear Corp. Nucleus' U.S. subsidiary. "They've been told by doctors that nothing can be done to help them. We need to educate the public about this implant." Sinclair believes that more success stories like Meier's will help spread the word. (Wharton 1986, 24)

* * *

Jason is one of eight children in the school's kindergarten/first grade class. He was recently featured in this year's United Way campaign film. The film was shown to corporate sponsors and portions of it have also aired as public service spots on television. "He's pretty typical of all the kids in his class. But they picked him because he was so cute," said Mary Beth Donze, Jason's teacher. (Karkabi 1988)

Other approaches have been to create advertising campaigns in print and television media. For example, a thirty-second television commercial for the Virginia Mason Medical Center in the United States and cost US$5,000 won advertising awards in the late 1980s. With no sound, and white type on a black screen, the commercial began,

> It's Valentine's Day at Virginia Mason [medical center]. A first grade teacher named Mrs. Roberta Ricketts is having an operation. She is totally deaf, unable to hear a single child's voice. But in less than five weeks, she'll go back into her classroom, wearing a computerized cochlear implant. And she won't believe her ears. . . . [The woman's photo appears along with a chorus of children's voices.] "Good morning Mrs. Ricketts. Welcome back, Mrs. Ricketts." Finally, one little girl asks in a hushed voice, "Can you hear me when I whisper?" (Updike 1988, 2)

THE REPRESENTATION OF, AND RESPONSE BY, DEAF PEOPLE

> The ultimate promise of any implant lies with deaf children. . . . If it can help them learn to speak, the cochlear implant could one day eliminate the isolated subculture of the deaf. (Mills 1985)

* * *

The article on Dr. William House's cochlear implants is another appalling example of ignorance by medical "experts" in regard to deaf culture. Contrary to the statement, "To many born deaf, the hearing world is threatening and alien," many deaf people view the hearing world as part of everyday living and as an exciting challenge to surmount barriers that are placed in our paths by those who, out of sheer ignorance, fear us. Our world is not of 'stony" silence but is a world filled with experience, truth and understanding. The deaf have a strong linguistic and cultural identity, not because we "feel safer in our environment," as Dr. House claims, but because we have a proud heritage. Would Dr. House lambaste black or Hispanic individuals, who after a long day of work with Caucasians, return to their homes and friends who may be of similar ethnic backgrounds and share certain experiences? Would he also say such individuals feel safer? The medical profession, including Dr. House, must learn that deafness is not just a medical condition but is also a viable cultural and linguistic entity that has its place in society. We are not alienated but it is individuals such as Dr. House who alienate us. (Miller 1985)

Twenty years after the publication of the two quotes above, and fifteen years since FDA approval was given, the number of child cochlear implant recipients to reach adolescence or early adulthood continues to grow. In the final part of this chapter, a sample of press articles reported in this study is analyzed for the view of deafness they construct and represent to the reader. In making this selection, articles that reflect one or the other of two world views or paradigms are included: either a medical view of deafness as a deficit or disability or a sociocultural view of deaf people as members of a cultural and linguistic minority. The first selection made is a series of three articles about Rory Osbrink, who received a cochlear implant at age four in 1980. More than twenty years later, a follow-up story appeared in the *Sacramento Bee* in which Rory discusses his opposition to childhood implantation. The second selection is a sample of articles on which a textual analysis is undertaken. After identifying the main "participants" in the text (in this case, deafness and cochlear implantation) and identifying the words directly associated with those "participants" from the text, one can clearly see the way in which deafness and cochlear implantation is represented in the texts.

The Story of Rory Osbrink

> Rory Osbrink had been deaf about a year when he ran out into the street and into the path of an oncoming fire engine. Rory, then 4, didn't hear the blaring siren. He didn't notice neighbors moving out of the way. He didn't hear his mother scream. The fire engine stopped 3 feet from where the Tustin youngster stood. Mary and Robert Osbrink had been agonizing for months about whether Rory should get a cochlear implant. . . . Rory's close call with the fire truck made the decision for them. (Downey 1987, B1)

Rory was the second child to be implanted through the House Ear Institute in Los Angeles. His parents described him as "making great strides" with his implant (Boutelle 1985, 8), and he was "considered a star of the implant program" (Downey 1987, B1). He had to be ordered to take the external processor off at bedtime, he "loves his implant so much," and he cried "I don't want to be deaf, I don't want to be deaf. . . . Fix it! Fix it!" after he jumped into a lake without realizing he was wearing the device (Downey 1987, B1).

In 2001, an article in the *Sacramento Bee* began:

> As a child, Rory Osbrink was a walking advertisement for the cochlear implant. Today, at 25, his device is turned off for good and Rory relies mostly on American sign language [sic], the vernacular of the deaf culture he has proudly joined. (Griffith 2001, 11)

As a child he became a "poster boy" for the cochlear implant: "His success was well-documented, and he was the star at events such as golf tournaments to raise money for research at the House Ear Institute" (Griffith 2001, 11). At sixteen, he stopped using the implant altogether. "Later, he explained to his parents that he had felt left out with the implant and that signed language made learning easier and more comfortable" (11). He is now opposed to childhood implantation but does not resent his parents for their decision. "Parents have a large role in decision-making, but they don't have a right to make uneducated decisions" (11).

Textual Analysis

To illustrate the representation of deafness in texts about cochlear implantation, I selected a second group of articles that include key statements related to the nature of deafness, Deaf people, or both.

I have identified "cochlear implantation" and "deafness" as the main "participants" in these texts and have grouped them as representing either a medical view of deafness or a sociocultural view of deafness. By listing the nouns associated with "cochlear implantation" and "deafness," a pattern of representation becomes visible (see table 5.1). This pattern shows the difference in perspectives taken toward the same topic and identifies the author's choices (as opposed to others that could have been made). Deafness, for example, is referred to by the hearing authors in ways that foreground isolation and fear. There is repeated reference to silence ("utter silence," "utterly silent world," "silent world," and "world of silence") and to the relentlessness of deafness ("permanent" and "without remedy"). This view of deafness stands in stark contrast to the representation by Deaf authors, who view deafness as "normal" and who foreground the sociocultural ("culture," "Deaf pride," "way of life," "shared world," "deaf history and values," "alliance," and "identity"). Similarly, the representation of cochlear implantation by hearing authors highlights a positive future ("medical breakthrough," "new ear," "new life," and "miraculous") whereas Deaf authors refer to its irrelevance and threat to their lives ("more like a hearing person at any cost").

The representation of "cochlear implantation" and "deafness" in these articles is further illustrated by listing the verbs with each topic (see table 5.2). Deafness, from a medical perspective, is identified with lack of hope ("condemned," "rely," "lost," "destined to be," "no hope," "dependent on") and inability to hear or lack of hearing attributes ("couldn't use the phone," "couldn't hear the television," "only babbling," "difficulty speaking") whereas implantation is associated with positive (mostly hearing) traits: hearing, understanding, talking, listening, being able to talk (similar to Deaf authors' use of positive actions associated with deafness: learn, develop, use, socialize, marry, hope, and want). Implantation, for Deaf authors, is linked to negative associations: "don't need," "is not worth," and "removes the right of the child."

Readers of these texts are positioned by (all) the authors in relation to cochlear implantation and deafness. Textual analysis enables the reader to see how the main topics have been represented by the author: what has been foregrounded and what has been excluded in the text.

As a result of this textual analysis, another difference between the medical and sociocultural perspectives has become evident: the idea of integrated versus distinct worlds. In the texts analyzed, reference to different "worlds" by hearing authors outnumbers those by Deaf authors 10 to 2. That is, there are ten occurrences of "world," "society," or "universe" in the articles by hearing authors whereas there are only two references by Deaf authors—one reference to "world"

Table 5.1. Descriptors Associated with Main Topics

Perspective	Descriptors associated with Deafness	Descriptors associated with Cochlear Implantation
Medical view of deafness	"permanent and without remedy" (Rabkin 1982, 13) "debilitating, isolated world of utter silence" (Dreyfuss 1985, 1) "profoundly deaf" (PR Newswire 1985a, 10) "[signed language was] the only way these children were able to communicate" (Ricks 1986, 1) "very lonely" (Wharton 1986, 24) "pretty scary" (Wharton 1986, 24) "things he lost" (Wharton 1986, 24) "utterly silent world" (Emmons 1988, 1) "silent world" (Dames 1989, n.p.) "world of silence" (Griffiths 1989, A11) "frustrated" (Murray 1989, 11)	"hearing universe" (Dreyfuss 1985, 1) "more sophisticated lip readers" (Emmons 1988, 1) "a new ear" (Edelson 1986, 3) "a new life" (Edelson 1986, 3) "in the hearing world with everyone else" (Scripps 1988, A1) "[the] only hope" (Murray 1989, 11) "no guarantee" (Tuck 1989a, J2) "medical breakthrough" (Dames 1989, n.p.) "nearly miraculous" (Dames 1989, n.p.) "artificial ear" (Saltus 1989, 27)
Sociocultural view of deafness	"normal" (Randal 1988a, 10) "full life using other forms of communication such as sign language" (Randal 1988a, 10)" "very angry" (Sydney Morning Herald 1988, 8) "sign language" (Sydney Morning Herald 1988, 8) "a culture that has no use for sound" (Saltus 1989, 27) "Deaf pride" (Saltus 1989, 27) "a way of life they espouse with pride" (Saltus 1989, 27) "normal" (Saltus 1989, 27) "shared world" (Saltus 1989, 27) "deaf history and values" (Saltus 1989, 27) "Deaf pride movement" (Saltus 1989, 27) "American Sign Language is my first language, English is my second" (Saltus 1989, 27) "powerful symbol of alliance among deaf people" (Saltus 1989, 27) "sense of identity" (Saltus 1989, 27)	"terrible threat" (Sydney Morning Herald 1988, 8) "more like a hearing a person at any cost" (Randal 1988a, 10) "irrelevant" (Saltus 1989, 27) "threat [to a way of life]" (Saltus 1989, 27) "medical agendas" (Saltus 1989, 27)

Table 5.2. Verb strings associated with the main topics

Perspective	Verb strings associated with Deafness	Verb strings associated with Cochlear Implantation
Medical view of deafness	"condemned to a world of silence" (Rabkin 1982, 13) "rely on sign language and lip-reading" (PR Newswire 1985a, 10) "lost" (Wharton 1986, 24) "couldn't use" (Wharton 1986, 24) "couldn't hear" (Wharton 1986, 24) "was destined to be in the deaf world forever" (Wharton 1986, 24) "communicating with hand signs" (Emmons 1988, 1) "crying" (Emmons 1988, 1) "laughing" (Emmons 1988, 1) "making only high-pitched babbling sounds" (Emmons 1988, 1) "hold back" (Emmons 1988, 1) "[has] difficulty speaking" (Dames 1989, 4S) "lived in silence" (Edelson 1986, 3) "no hope of talking properly" (Scripps 1988, A1) "not responding" (Murray 1989, 11) "start to cry" (Murray 1989, 11) "suffer in silence" (Tuck 1989a, J2) "is dependent on sign language" (Tuck 1989a, J2) "stop talking" (Tuck 1989a, J2)	"liberates" (Dreyfuss 1985, 1) "hearing" (Ricks 1986, 1) "provides" (Ricks 1986, 1) "[go] back to work" (Thomas 1986, 3) "live a 'close to normal' life" (Thomas 1986, 3) "studies" (Wharton 1986, 24) "can understand ... without ... a sign-language interpreter" (Wharton 1986, 24) "talks" (Wharton 1986, 24) "listens to birds sing" (Wharton 1986, 24) "has gained back" (Wharton 1986, 24) "They're back to the hearing world" (Baker 1988, 4) "break free" (Emmons 1988, 1) "abandon hand signs" (Emmons 1988, 1) "becoming a part of mainstream society" (Emmons 1988, 1) "hear" (Dames 1989, n.p.) "back in the hearing community" (Griffiths 1989, A11) "learned to read lips" (Tuck 1989a, J2) "able to talk" (Tuck 1989a, J2)

Sociocultural view of deafness	"grew up in a Deaf family" (Randal 1988a, 10) "has no interest in an implant" (Randal 1988a, 10) "learned to adjust" (Randal 1988a, 10) "develop alternative warning systems" (Randal 1988a, 10) "use our eyes more" (Randal 1988a, 10) "never heard" (Randal 1988a, 10) "don't miss it" (Randal 1988a, 10) "actively opposed" (Saltus 1989, 27) "born deaf" (Saltus 1989, 27) "use American Sign Language" (Saltus 1989, 27) "speaking in American Sign Language" (Saltus 1989, 27) "socialize together, marry each other" (Saltus 1989, 27) "hoped her baby would be born deaf" (Saltus 1989, 27) "want my daughter to be like me, to be deaf" (Saltus 1989, 27) "belong to the Deaf community" (Sydney Morning Herald 1988, 8)	"Don't need" (Randal 1988a, 10) "is not worth the trouble" (Randal 1988a, 10) "[signals that] hearing is preferable to deafness" (Saltus 1989, 27) "view with suspicion" (Saltus 1989, 27) "encourage the totally deaf to learn to speak" (Saltus 1989, 27) "fit into their world" (Saltus 1989, 27) "moves the right of the child" (Sydney Morning Herald 1988, 8)

and one to "shared world." A medical perspective of deafness as a deficit or disability constructs a Deaf-World that is isolated, closed, and removed from "mainstream society." Hearing authors state that implantation

- "lets deaf children enter [the] world of hearing" (Ricks 1986, 1);
- enables a deaf person to "participate in the hearing world" (Griffiths 1989, 1);
- helps return them "back to the hearing world" (Baker 1988, 4);
- enables them to "become a part of the hearing world" (Griffiths 1989, 1);
- allows "a world that wouldn't exist" without an implant (Dreyfuss 1985, 1).

Saltus (1989) describes the two views: "[It] depends on whether you see a hearing-impaired person as part of the world at large, or part of a closed society where you exist with your own kind" (27). An alternate view is to consider the universe as a shared, diverse world that includes various communities, subcultures, and minority groups.

AFTERWORD

This chapter has taken an historical approach, using the advantage of hindsight to view the claims for implantation made during the 1980s and early 1990s, a crucial period in which cochlear implantation was being tried on an experimental basis and later approved for use with adults and children. One should not assume, however, that the issues identified in the analysis of articles published in the first decade of media representation of cochlear implantation are no longer relevant. Key themes identified in the articles analyzed in this chapter—cochlear implantation as miracle cure, charitable donations to finance implantation, unpredictability of outcomes, and views of normalcy—are still evident in press articles today. For example, the word *miracle* is still closely associated with implantation, as illustrated by the following text, published in the United Kingdom in 2005 (*Peterborough Evening Telegraph* 2005, 24):

> One-year-old Ava was born profoundly deaf. Now, only the miracle of modern medical science will help her hear the sound of her mother's voice for the first time. Ava, who had her first birthday party last week, will be one of the youngest children in the country to have a hi-tech implant inserted in her ear. Already Zara . . . is excited that her daughter will be freed from a world of silence.

The word *miracle* again appeared recently in an Australian article (Rao 2005, 18): "Braithe French [age three years] has not blurted out his first word or taken his first step yet, but he is still a 'miracle' in his parents' eyes." This article also provides evidence of the continuing themes of charity and uncertain outcomes:

> A . . . cochlear implant costs nothing for the recipient but costs the charity $60,000 [Australian dollars] in all to put each child it deals with through its hearing program. "Luckily he was eligible for a cochlear implant, which we couldn't afford," said Mrs. French [the child's mother].

Professor Bill Gibson [director of the Sydney Cochlear Implant Centre] said he was hopeful that Braithe's implant would prove a success, although he was cautious about his optimism. "It's only early days," he said. (Rao 2005, 18)

The view of "normalcy" is also used in connection with implantation (and here, is used with *miracle*):

But the *miracle* of cochlear implants and the help of staff at the Shepherd Centre [Sydney] means Taylor [age four or five years] will be starting at a mainstream primary school on January 31, at the same age and ability level as her peers. She had a bad start to life—"to [now] be able to speak and listen and play just as a normal child is wonderful," Taylor's mother Jenny said. "When you get told your child is deaf you don't know what their life is going to be like." Aged one, Taylor received a cochlear implant. It was switched on two weeks later. "It was just magical, her eyes lit up," Mrs. Johnston said. Mrs. Johnston and Taylor visited the Shepherd Centre for one hour each week in a bid to teach Taylor to talk and listen *like non-hearing impaired children*. The centre runs one-on-one lessons with children and their parents as well as a playgroup that includes both *hearing capable and hearing impaired* children. "Without the intervention of the Shepherd Centre Taylor wouldn't be going to a mainstream school, I don't think," Mrs. Johnston said. Enrolling Taylor into a mainstream school was important to her parents, who wanted their daughter to live as much of a *normal* life as possible. "It was very important because I didn't want her to be treated differently, I wanted her to be treated as part of a *normal* school background," Mrs. Johnston said. (Trenwith 2005, 7, emphasis added)

U.S. Food and Drug Administration data from 2005 indicated there were almost 100,000 implant recipients worldwide. Since researching the data for this chapter, a medical and deficit representation of deafness continues to dominate the pages of the daily press. Most recently, bilateral implantation has become an emerging trend, one that is heralded as having the potential—alongside anticipated improvements in auditory outcomes—to double manufacturers' profits (Australian Associated Press, 2006).

REFERENCES

Associated Press. 1985. New implant opens world of sound for deaf people. *Los Angeles Times*. March 24, 2–3.

Australian Associated Press. 2006. Bilateral ear implants 'emerging trend.' September 22.

Baker, B. 1988. "Electronic inner ear" gives shower of noise. *Los Angeles Times*, March 14, Metro section, 4.

The Baton Rouge Sunday Advocate. 1989. Ear implant studied. February 26, E3.

Berg, P. 1985a. Hearing rediscovered: PBS looks at the cochlear implant. *The Washington Post*, May 1, H20.

———. 1985b. Cutting edge brain difference found between right- and left-handed people. *The Washington Post*, September 18, H5.

———. 1985c. News and notes about health. *The Washington Post*, March 20, H5.

Boutelle, J. 1985. The Irvine Company's new generation. *Orange County Business Journal*, September, 8(9): Section 1, 8.

Bown, B. G. 1989. TV celebs pitch in to help deaf girl. *Atlanta Journal and Constitution*, August 18, J06.

Brody, L. 1988. Device opens world of sound for 5-year-old. *St. Petersburg Times*, August 1, 1 and 5.

Brown, M. 1989. Fingers do the talking—hearing aid and lip reading. *The Sunday Times*, July 30.

Bruckheim, A. 1987. "Tropical" rash isn't serious. *Chicago Tribune*, March 16, 8.

Business Wire. 1989. Cochlear Corp. acquires 3M cochlear implant business. August 15, 8.

Cameron, D., and Y. Steinhauer. 1987. First, waiting for the miracle. *Sydney Morning Herald*, September 19, 1.

Canada News-Wire. 1989. Rotary Club of Vancouver—Bike-a-thon. July 8.

Chase, M. 1984a. Body shop: firm that developed artificial heart seeks to build bionic market. *The Wall Street Journal*, July 24.

———. 1984b. Kolff "artificial ear" is implanted in man by surgeons in Utah. *The Wall Street Journal*, April 11.

Chicago Tribune. 1986. New implant buoys hope for deaf. August 17, 3.

Cochlear Corporation. 2005. *Cochlear 2005 Annual Report*. http://www.cochlear.com/PDFs/AR05_editorial.pdf (accessed January 13, 2006).

Dames, J. 1989. Northwest plaza being transformed into a princely ballroom. *St. Louis Post-Dispatch*, July 23, 4S (late five star edition).

Downey, C. 1987. Sounds from silence. Cochlear implant: Letting in world of noise. *The Orange County Register*, April 20, Metro section, 1.

Dreyfuss, J. 1985. Implant liberates the deaf from silence. *Los Angeles Times*, January 29, View section, 1.

Edelson, E. 1986. New body parts offer hope for the impaired. *The Dallas Morning News*, December 15, Today section, 3.

Emmons, S. 1988. Ian's world may be silent, but it's not quiet. *Los Angeles Times*, May 29, Metro section, 1.

Feldman, C. 1985. Experimental implant rescues man from years of deafness. *Houston Chronicle*, August 18, 5.

Galarneau, J. 1988. Regaining a sense of the world: Cochlear implant patient reclaims some sounds he once heard. *St. Petersburg Times*, June 12, 1; 3; 7.

Gindick, T. 1985. When Dr. Victor Goodhill talks ears, people listen. *Los Angeles Times*, November 5, View section, 1.

Griffith, D. 2001. A strong belief in going without cochlear implant. *The Sacramento Bee*, December 30, A11.

Griffiths, J. 1989. Jury's out on hearing device: Soundness of cochlear implant remains open to question. *The Evening News Harrisburg*, May 8, C1.

HealthWeek. 1988. Intrapreneurs: Innovation from within. November 14, 219.

Immen, W. 1984. Man given ear implant able to detect sound after 50 years silence. *The Globe and Mail*, August 13, M7.

Johnson, G. T. 1985. Ear implants not for all hearing loss patients. *Chicago Tribune*, May 15, 7.

Karkabi, B. 1988. School for deaf children teaches how to listen, speak. *Houston Chronicle*, September 27, 1.

Kavanagh, J. 1988. Mike Hirshorn—Nucleus Group Technology. *Business Review Weekly*, December 9, 62.

Komesaroff, L. 2002. Applying social critical literacy theory to deaf education. *Australian Journal of Language and Literacy*, 252:37–46.

Kotulak, R., and J. Van. 1987. Olive oil may lower your blood pressure. *Chicago Tribune*, June 28, 5.

Lufkin, L. 1988. '90s: Space chats and romance. A brave new decade filled with fun. *The San Francisco Chronicle*, August 24, B3.

Luke, A. 2000. Critical literacy in Australia: A matter of context and standpoint. *Journal of Adolescent & Adult Literacy*, 43 (5):448–61.

Lumby, C. 1989. And here is to love, life, peace and lots of joy. *Sydney Morning Herald*, December 11, 17.

Mcadam, M., and J. Eyers. 2004. *The Financial Review*. U.S. probe deals Cochlear resounding blow. March 13.

Miller, B. 1985. Culture of the deaf. *Los Angeles Times*, February 17, View section, 19.

Mills, D. 1984. FDA clears device giving deaf people awareness of sound: 3M, the product's marketer, estimates 200,000 in U.S. could have it implanted. *The Wall Street Journal*, November 30.

———. 1985. Many deaf prefer static to silence, but others expected to hear Beethoven. *The Wall Street Journal*, February 21.

Millsap, J. 1987. Implant may give deaf girl chance to learn speech. *Houston Chronicle*, June 9, 16.

Molotsky, I. 1984. Food and Drug Administration approves electronic ear implant that could . . . *New York Times*, November 30, Section 1, 1.

Murray, M. 1989. Ear implant opens new world for deaf. *The Toronto Star*, May 25, 11.

The Observer. The big issue: Abuse of deaf children: Why it is so hard for the hard of hearing, March 27, Letters section.

The Omaha World-Herald. 1986. Davenport Hospital performing implants for the profoundly deaf. September 18.

———. 1987. Implants researched in Iowa: Devices help children hear at last. October 5.

O'Neill, C. 1985. How and why? *Washington Post*, August 28, H18.

Pemberton-Reid, F. R. 1987. Friends raise money to help deaf boy hear. *Star-Tribune*, June 11, Y1.

Perlman, D. 1985. Implant developed at UC: Hearing device for the totally deaf. *The San Francisco Chronicle*, March 8, 3.

Peterborough Evening Telegraph. 2005. Hearing hope for baby Ava. March 30, Health section, 24.

Petit, C. 1987. Success with devices for deaf. *The San Francisco Chronicle*, December 1, A24.

Pollack, A. 1988. Electronic nerves: Scientific advances hold new promise for physically impaired. *New York Times*, January 9, D1.

Porco, D. L. 1985. Culture of the deaf. *Los Angeles Times*, February 17.

Power, D. 2005. Models of deafness: Cochlear implants in the Australian daily press. *The Journal of Deaf Studies and Deaf Education*, 104:451–59.

Prior, N. 1988. Alex's new ear is fun, but it gets stuck to the fridge. *Sydney Morning Herald*, August 2, 2.

PR Newswire. 1985a. College student's hearing restored by surgically implanted hearing device. December 4.

———. 1985b. Symbion tests Ineraid artificial-ear. July 22.

Rabkin, B. 1982. Implant gives limited hearing to woman. *The Globe and Mail*, November 24, 13.

Randal, J. E. 1988a. In the deaf community, promise and suspicion. *The Washington Post*, May 10, Health section, 10.

———. 1988b. Your health: Implants for the hearing-impaired. *Newsday*, May 24, 11.

Rao, S. 2005. Brave Braithe hears at last. *Daily Telegraph*, January 26, O18.

Ricks, D. 1986. Implant lets deaf children enter world of hearing. *Los Angeles Times*, March 2, Metro section, 1.

Roan, S. 1989. Implants help the deaf perceive sound. *The Orange County Register*, August 24, D6.

Saltus, R. 1989. Returning to the world of sound: Cochlear implants, the closest thing to artificial ears, proving helpful to more and more people. *The Boston Globe*, July 10, 27.

Schroer, J. 1987. A big hospital in a small space: Now age 30, doctors still thrive on marketing specialty medical services. *The Orange County Register*, February 24, O9.

Scripps, H. 1988. $17,000 hearing aid: 3-year-old deaf girl's silent world now beeping by computer. *The Evening News Harrisburg*, March 22, A1.

The Seattle Times. 1985. Device lets deaf hear, but how? June 2, A14.

———. 1988. Boy, 3, to have implant surgery; cost is a worry. August 1, B4.

Shaw, R. 1985. Scherer-Storz: Atlanta's alpine connection. *Business Atlanta*, May 1, 98.

Signor, R. 1989. Sound for Sally: Experimental surgery lets a deaf 17-year-old hear some sounds. *St. Louis Post-Dispatch*, September 30, D1.

Slee, A. 1987. Lack of funds threatens bionic ear development. *Sydney Morning Herald*, August 8, 13.

Smollar, D. 1986. New implant surgery gives hearing back to the deaf. *Los Angeles Times*, February 4, Metro section, 5.

Special Correspondent. 1987. Science report: Electronic takeover when the nerves fail. *The Times*, December 26.

Stuart, A. 1988. Good medicine innovations offer new help for old problems. *Chicago Tribune*, June 12, Tempo section, 7.

Sun Herald. 1988. The eye. October 30, 96.

Sydney Morning Herald. 1988. Aust ear implant set to help deaf children. May 19, 8.

Thomas, C. 1986. Government won't pay for mother's $11,000 "bionic ear." *Sydney Morning Herald*, November 21, 3.

———. 1987. Hospital's savings earn bionic ears for 10. *Sydney Morning Herald*, November 21, 4.

Thompson, L. 1985. Spare parts. *The Washington Post*, January 23, Health section, 12.

Times Wire Services. 1987. Researchers announce new aid for deaf. *Los Angeles Times*, December 1.

Trenwith, C. 2005. Taylor off to school—hear, hear! *Illawarra Mercury*, January 18, 7.

Tuck, A. D. 1989a. Little Nikki's world is silent no more: 6-year-old's hearing restored with surgery. *Atlanta Journal and Constitution*, November 25, J2.

———. 1989b. Girl's ear-implant surgery a success: Nikki, 6, recovering from first step toward regaining her hearing. *Atlanta Journal and Constitution*, October 12, J2.

Updike, R. 1988. John Brown & Partners Inc: Creativity is credo for this risk-taking advertising agency. *The Seattle Times*, June 6, B2.

Van, J. 1987. Device may help hearing-impaired: Transmitter in skull bypasses nature's sound. *Chicago Tribune*, September 17.

Walker, L. A. 1987. Listen up: Your ears are more precious than you think. *Chicago Tribune*, March 4, Style section, 16.

Wall Street Journal. 2002. Meningitis cases are found among ear-implant patients. July 26, A1.

Wharton, D. 1986. "I can hear birds, wind, rain!" Experimental aural implant holds hope for some deaf. *Los Angeles Times*, June 5, View section, 24.

United Press International. 1985. Every noise is a pleasure to once-deaf man. *Houston Chronicle*, September 25.

U.S.A Today. 1987. Colorado. June 11, A06.

6

THE PSYCHOSOCIAL DEVELOPMENT OF DEAF CHILDREN WITH COCHLEAR IMPLANTS

Gunilla Preisler

This chapter discusses the psychosocial situation for deaf children with cochlear implants from multiple perspectives: the parents' perspective, the teachers' perspective, and the children's perspective. It considers results from international research and a recent Swedish longitudinal study that (a) indicate problems if communication and education for children with implants is based only on speech and (b) suggest that a cochlear implant cannot replace using sign language, but it can facilitate everyday life in hearing families.

Nearly fifteen years have passed since the first deaf child in Sweden received a cochlear implant. Today, almost 90 percent of deaf children are implanted each year, many of them bilaterally. What do we now know about the effects of the implant on the life conditions of these children? Until the mid-1970s, deaf children predominantly received an oral education in most countries around the world. The implications of this practice were that being deaf was understood as being disabled and that the opportunity to obtain good school results and therefore take part in the wider society was limited (Gregory 2002). Has improved hearing ability, the case for most children receiving an implant, given them increased opportunities to use and understand speech as well as to take part in cultural and social activities with hearing people? Do they now have a better quality of life?

These questions raise an important methodological issue for researchers, namely, how to measure quality of life in these children. Most deaf children who receive an implant today, receive it at an early age. Therefore, it is not possible for them either to compare what it was like to live without an implant or to imagine what it would have been like. One way of addressing this problem is to make comparisons between deaf children with implants and deaf children of similar age and in similar circumstance who do not have implants. However, it is not easy to find a group of deaf children without implants that is comparable with a group of children with cochlear implants in all relevant aspects other than the implant. A number of comparative studies between children with cochlear implants and those using other technical devices have been made with respect to the outcomes on speech perception and speech production tests (see, for example, Geers and Moog 1994; Miyamoto et al. 1995; Meyer et al. 1998; Allen, Nikolopoulos, and O'Donoghue 1998; Svirsky et al. 2000). However, it has been difficult to draw valid conclusions from these studies because baseline information (on measures of hearing status, language ability, or other related variables such as the families' level of education or socioeconomic status) that would determine the degree of comparability between the groups before those in the implant group received their implants is seldom or never made available (Spencer and Marschark 2003).

The studies mentioned above indicated that the children made progress with the implant. However, that progress—discriminating certain target words or being able to utter single words and simple sentences—is not sufficient when one wants to take part in social activities with others. In many studies, the child's auditory development is mistaken for language ability (Blamey et al. 2001). Blume (2002) made a review of studies on quality of life in adults and children. He found the studies indicated that there were positive effects of implantation. He also found that the children themselves were not involved in the studies. Either experts (physicians and researchers) or parents (who responded on behalf of the child) decided what important improvements were made after implantation. Measurement of quality of life with respect to cochlear implants has primarily concerned the costs and benefits of the procedure (see O'Neill et al. 2001). These studies adopted a dominant societal or hearing perspective. To date, there have been no studies from the perspective of deaf children themselves (Blume 2002).

In this chapter, I intend to shed light on the children's psychosocial situation, not only from a societal or hearing perspective (mainly represented by parents and teachers) but also from the children's own perspective. I use the term psychosocial to mean the child's potential and ability to initiate and comprehend communication with others. Reciprocity, mutual understanding, and shared meaning are regarded as important prerequisites for well-functioning psychosocial development. The children's language, play, and interactions will be regarded as important markers of psychosocial developmental processes.

THEORETICAL BACKGROUND

Studies of infant development have shown that a child is socially active from the first minutes of life and that learning takes places in interaction with others in meaningful contexts. Newborns can imitate expressions of the face, hands, or voice of another person (Kugiumutzakis 1998; Nadel et al. 1999). According to Trevarthen (2004), these results indicate that infants are ready to pick up the motives of other people. Today, there is also physiological evidence of an innate ability to understand another's motives. Humans have been found to be equipped with cells in the cortex that have neural mirroring elements. These appear to anticipate the evolution of imitations that make learning of human speech and language possible (Rizzolatti and Arbib 1998).

To learn to communicate, a child must be engaged in repeated and habitual social exchanges where the child and the caregiver are intimately involved in constructing reality through finely tuned relationships (MacDonald and Carroll 1994). In encounters with others—caregivers and members of the family and, later on, peers and other adults—the child gradually develops a sense of self in relation to not only the psychosocial but also the physical world (Stern 2000). Depending on how these encounters develop, the child will create an inner image of self with others. Traditional developmental psychology has been formed on the idea of the child as an individual constructor of meaning and knowledge. In contrast, interdisciplinary research has clearly shown that developmental processes such as language learning and interpersonal communication involve both the caregiver and the child in active roles during the interaction (Fogel 1993; Tronick 1998; Stern 2000; Trevarthen 2004). But that interactive circle must be widened.

Parents are part of a cultural context, and they meet with other parents and professionals who express the same or other values and ideas. Like parents of any child, the way that parents of children with functional disabilities interact with their children is dependent on a variety of factors. How support systems and habilitation are managed and how parents experience this management are important variables for the future well-being of the child and family. Societal attitudes toward children with functional disabilities can influence the way parents look on their children's potential to develop.

Before parents decide whether their child is going to have an implant, they receive information from various formal and informal sources. Even if they get information from magazines, the Internet, friends, parents, or neighbors, the multidisciplinary team members, particularly the surgeons, are usually the first professionals to give parents detailed information about what it means for a child to have a cochlear implant (Kluwin and Stewart 2000; Preisler, Tvingstedt, and Ahlström 2002). To study what the members of these teams themselves thought about cochlear implants, three researchers, Ahlström, Preisler, and Tvingstedt, conducted interviews in 1995 with twenty-two members of multidisciplinary teams at two different hospitals in Sweden where the first operations in that country were made. One goal of the interviews was to learn about the discourse about deafness within these two teams as part of a continuing longitudinal psychosocial follow-up study of children with cochlear implants (Preisler, Ahlström, and Tvingstedt 1997; Preisler, Tvingstedt, and Ahlström 1999, 2002, 2003, 2005; Ahlström, Tvingstedt, and Preisler 1999; Tvingstedt, Preisler, and Ahlström 1999, 2000, 2001, 2003; Preisler 2001). It turned out that knowledge of and earlier contact with children in general, and deaf children in particular, was sparse among the members of the two teams, although many had experience working with hard of hearing adults.

In 1981, the Swedish government officially declared Swedish Sign Language as the language of the deaf community; consequently, special schools now attempt to educate deaf children bilingually in Swedish Sign Language, written Swedish and, whenever possible, spoken Swedish. In 2000, the Swedish National Board of Health and Welfare formulated a policy that sign language communication should be established between the child and his or her family before cochlear implantation was performed (2000, 43). Therefore, at the time of the study's interviews, Swedish Sign Language was the official language to be used with all deaf children, with or without an implant. Among the team members, only one person was considered by her colleagues to have a good command of Swedish Sign Language. Among the others, knowledge of sign language was limited. Their attitude to sign language use, on the surface, appeared positive. However, many of the team members considered deaf people as belonging to a minority group in society, with deaf children living in a restricted world that they would have to leave when they grew older and started their working lives. Isolation and dependence were considered possible and very likely consequences of a hearing impairment. The medico-technical members of both teams, in particular, claimed that the use of a cochlear implant would enhance the possibility of a deaf child gradually being able to speak and hear, even if the team could guarantee parents only that the implant would enable the perception of environmental sounds.

Parental Perspectives on Choosing a Cochlear Implant for Their Child

In the Swedish longitudinal study, twenty-two children who were born between 1990 and 1994 and who received cochlear implants before 1996 were followed from preschool age up to the first years of school. The children belong to the first generation of children in Sweden who have received a cochlear implant. Eleven girls and eleven boys took part in the study. The children were between the ages of one year eleven months and four years ten months at the time of implantation, with a mean age of three years and five months. At the end of the study, the children had worn their implants for a period of between five and almost seven and a half years.

The parents were interviewed about their opinion of the child's psychosocial situation. The first interviews were conducted when the children were of preschool age, the second before the children started school, and the third when the children had attended school between one and four years (Preisler, Tvingstedt, and Ahlström 1999). In the first interview, all the parents declared that Swedish Sign Language was the child's first language and that the children were to be looked on as deaf even after the operation. Six children were postlingually deaf and had some proficiency in spoken Swedish before becoming deaf. According to their parents, these children were also in need of sign language to fully take part in dialogues. All the parents maintained that their key motive for the operation was to increase the possibility that the child would become bilingual. Over time, as the parents perceived their child's proficiency in speech perception and increased speech production, less sign language communication was used. But as soon as the child needed a detailed explanation of some phenomena, when misunderstandings occurred, or when there was conflict, sign language was considered necessary (Tvingstedt, Preisler, and Ahlström 1999).

By the final interview, when the children had worn their implants between five years and seven years five months, the parents said that sign language was rarely used in the family. Most of the children were considered capable of participating in everyday conversations in the home. However, the parents still experienced difficulty when discussing complicated matters because the children's oral vocabulary as well as their ability to understand concepts and word meaning were limited. The children had difficulty articulating many words, which made it difficult for adults outside the family to understand their speech. All parents, regardless of which school their child attended, maintained the importance of sign language when explaining complicated, abstract, especially important, or new concepts (Preisler, Tvingstedt, and Ahlström 2003).

Patterns of Parent-Child Interaction in the Home Setting

The researchers visited the children at home every third month of the study and, during the visits, made video recordings in natural interactional settings with parents and siblings. Altogether, they made seventy-two recordings and direct observations. The first video recordings in the children's homes, soon after implantation, provided evidence that the parents and children mainly communicated in sign language or by using signs in combination with other nonverbal means of communication (Tvingstedt, Preisler, and Ahlström 1999). In more than half the families, the sign language communication was considered to be well functioning; in the others, less so. The use of signs was the natural basis for communication in most families. Even those parents who used speech still included sign communication. These observations were well in accordance with the parents' own statements in the interviews.

As time passed, all twenty-two parents in the study began to introduce more spoken language when communicating with their child. A consequence of this shift was that the parents were not paying the same degree of attention to establishing eye-to-eye contact with their child before starting to communicate as they had done at the start of the study. This change affected the pattern of turn taking and resulted in dialogue that was often disrupted, resulting in misunderstanding. When more speech was introduced, the communication could result in the parent using speech and the child using sign language and single spoken words. When the parents did not demand speech production from the child, when they were using speech as input, the resulting interaction was often smooth, without disruption or misunderstanding.

Toward the end of the preschool period, most of the children could take part in simple spoken dialogues in the family setting. They used some words or responded appropriately to their parent's speech by using nonverbal means of communication such as head nods or pointing. A characteristic of these interactions was that the topic of conversation was well known and the content was about the here and now. According to the parents, simple daily conversations in the family had been facilitated by the child's implantation. An important finding was that the children with the most developed oral language also had well-developed sign language. They were used to understanding and to being understood.

The parents' way of communicating with their children varied; the different styles used could be characterized as (a) an adult-centered, directive way of communicating or (b) a child-centered, supportive style (Barnes et al. 1983; Hoff-Ginsberg and Schatz 1982; Moseley 1990). When the parents used a more adult-centered and directive communicative style, the dialogue between the children and parents was generally short, often with only one turn being taken. When using a more child-centered communicative style, the conversations could develop into extensive dialogues with each speaker taking many turns. A feature of this style of communication was that the parents expanded on the subject in relation to the child's interests and utterances. In some cases with older children, these dialogues developed into the kind of narratives that are a part of the life stories children create. Being able to create an autobiographic narrative is an essential aspect of the child's development of identity and sense of self (Stern 2000).

PATTERNS OF INTERACTION IN THE PRESCHOOL SETTING

When the children entered the study, eight of the twenty-two children attended preschools for deaf children where Swedish Sign Language was used, and ten attended preschools for deaf and hard of hearing children where signs and speech were used simultaneously. Four children were mainstreamed into regular pre-schools for hearing children. The children were visited regularly during a two-year period, and the researchers made fifty-seven video recordings in natural interactional settings. When analyzing the interaction between teachers and children as well as between the children with cochlear implants and their peers, Ahlström, Tvingstedt, and Preisler (1999) focused on three different play activities in each of the preschool settings. In the preschools for deaf children where Swedish Sign Language was used, the main part of the video recorded interactions comprised a variety of structured adult-initiated activities such as meal times, game playing, storytelling, and so on. The conversations registered in these contexts were primarily between teacher and child. The communicative style of the teachers varied. Some used an adult-centered, directive style in some situations whereas others used a more child-centered, supportive communicative style. The level of linguistic activity was high, and fantasy and storytelling frequently occurred. When communicating with one another, the children used sign language, and the content of their dialogue could be considered age appropriate. They discussed events in the here and now and events in the future or past. The older children could also share fantasies, and symbolic play was observed among the deaf children (Jorup and Preisler 2001).

In the preschools for deaf and hard of hearing children, the implanted child was often the only deaf child in the group or the only child with a cochlear implant. Observations showed that sign-supported speech was the main communication approach used between the teachers and children. There were also instances when only sign language or only speech was used. The same phenomenon that occurred in the home environment was observed in the preschool setting. When teachers used speech only or sign-supported speech, they did not always ensure they had first established eye contact with the children. Thus, the children were not always aware they were being addressed, and misunderstandings occurred. The more speech the teachers used, the more uncertain the communication. If the context was clearly defined and the children knew what was expected from them, they could manage to take simple instructions in spoken language. The main communicative means used between the deaf child with a cochlear implant and children who did not know sign language were those of pointing, gestures, eye contact, and body movement. The communication was at a concrete and pre-symbolic level.

The four children in mainstream preschools were observed undertaking the same type of activities as had the children in the other preschool settings. However, symbolic communication between the hearing children and the deaf child during the video recorded interactions was not registered. Opportunities for the deaf child to take part in dialogue with his or her peers were limited. Instead, the deaf child interacted mostly with adults, particularly signing adults if one was present, and this adult often took on the role of interpreter both for the children and other adults. The deaf child was occasionally observed to take part in the hearing children's play but only in noncommunicative roles. The teachers working in general educational preschools had no prior experience of deaf or hard of hearing children, but considered the situation for the child with a cochlear implant as satisfactory. They seldom witnessed the child being involved in conflict or being harassed by other children, a matter of concern for teachers and parents before the child started preschool.

THE SCHOOL EXPERIENCE

As the children grew older, half the children attended special schools for deaf and hard of hearing students, and half attended general classes at the local school. The longitudinal study looked at this situation from the perspectives of the parents and teachers as well as considered the resulting interaction patterns that developed.

The Children's School Situation—From the Parents' Perspective

When the children in the study started school, the parents were asked about different aspects of their child's education (Preisler, Tvingstedt, and Ahlström 2003). The results showed that almost all parents expressed satisfaction with their choice of school placement for their child. These results are similar to the findings in the Archbold and colleagues (2002) study about parents' perception of their child's situation three years after implantation; however, in the Swedish study, the parents of children in regular schools believed the situation could have been improved if their child had received more personal support, if the support given had been of a different nature, and if the educational setting had been better adapted to the child's needs.

   The parents of children in the special schools expressed satisfaction with the school setting. They maintained that their child received an adequate education from which their child could profit. They were not content, however, with the status of speech in the special schools and wanted more speech training as part of the curriculum. The parents of the children in general educational classes were aware of their child's difficulty discriminating speech in a noisy environment and understanding words and meanings, which made it hard for them to understand information given by the teachers. They still preferred this school setting because they did not want to move or let their child live away from home. It turned out that the two main factors explaining choice of school were distance from the special school and prior educational placement at preschool. Parents who lived close enough to a special school to have their children commute and whose children had attended special preschool education chose the special school; others chose general education classes. For most parents in the Swedish study, moving the family to a new residential area or allowing their child to attend boarding school was not an attractive alternative (Tvingstedt, Preisler, and Ahlström 2003).

   Peer interaction was also a matter of concern for all parents in the Swedish study regardless of which school setting their child attended. Most of the children in general educational classes were boys, and they often took part in physical activities, that is, mostly nonverbal activities. In these situations, they could manage quite well with hearing peers. Similar results have been obtained in a study by Martin and Bat-Chava (2003). Deaf boys' relationships with hearing peers benefited mostly from the boys' ability to perform well in sports. According to the parents of children in general education classes in the Swedish longitudinal study, their children had few close friends in or outside school with whom they could communicate. In most cases, the children in the special schools had friends at the school or in their class with whom they could communicate. But the children in general education classes had few if any friends outside school (Preisler, Tvingstedt, and Ahlström 2003).

The Children's School Situation—From the Teachers' Perspective

Thirteen teachers working in the special schools were interviewed in the Swedish longitudinal study (Preisler, Tvingstedt, and Ahlström 2003). Most teachers had more than thirty years of experience in deaf education; many also had academic degrees in Swedish Sign Language, interpreting, or both. The teachers at special schools maintained that placement in their type of school was appropriate for children with cochlear implants because the children's perception and production of speech was limited and because they were not considered able to profit from an education in spoken Swedish. In some cases, the children's sign language proficiency was limited, which caused some educational problems. In three cases, there was no doubt about the choice of school placement because the children no longer used their implants. The teachers concluded in two of these cases that the implant was no longer used because the child was unable to pay attention to the auditory input, and they concluded in one case that technical deficiencies of the implant had led to its disuse. The teachers of the children in both the regular and special school settings reported a wide variation in the children's knowledge and learning capacities. These differences partly covaried with language capacity. Otherwise, they maintained that these children performed in much the same way as any other deaf child.

Interviews were conducted with twelve teachers in general education classes soon after the children had started school (Preisler, Tvingstedt, and Ahlström 2003). Most of these teachers had been teaching for between twenty-five and thirty-five years. Their initial opinion was that the present school situation was adequate for a child with a cochlear implant. When asked more specifically about deafness, deaf children, and cochlear implantation, their knowledge and prior experience of deaf children's situations was practically nonexistent. Their expectations of the children's learning potential and competence was initially very low, but when the children started school, the teachers were impressed and surprised at how well they could adapt to the school situation with other hearing pupils (Preisler, Tvingstedt, and Ahlström 2003).

However, after two or three years of experience with a child with a cochlear implant in their classes, the teachers in the general education classes were aware of the difficulties in providing adequate educational stimulation to the child. Lack of resources, lack of knowledge and support, and class size put great demands on the teachers. They maintained that the child had to adapt to the conditions in a class with hearing pupils and pointed out that they could not perform "miracles." The adaptation made to the regular classroom was to employ a teacher assistant who used Swedish Sign Language. During the first school year, most of the deaf children took part in classes with all the pupils present, but as time passed, many of them spent more time with the teacher assistant, receiving individual tutoring and spending less time in the regular classroom. Another problem was that the teachers were not always aware of the child's level of performance.

Because the child and the assistant worked so closely together, it was not always clear whether it was the assistant or the child who had completed a particular task.

Interviews with seven teacher assistants showed that they had received little information in advance of the child's placement at the school about how to assist a child with a cochlear implant in the general education classroom. They were generally given no time for preparing lessons and seldom knew what the classroom teacher intended to teach on any particular day. They were often expected to interpret what the teacher said in the classroom, despite the fact that several of them had limited sign language competence, as did a number of the children with cochlear implants. There were many similarities between the parents' and teachers' assessments of the same child's capabilities and difficulties. Both teachers and parents were aware of what the child was good at and what improvements could be accomplished.

Patterns of Interaction in the Classroom

To shed light on the school situation Preisler, Tvingstedt, and Ahlström (forthcoming) made video recordings in the classrooms of the oldest children over a two-year period and in the settings for the youngest children over a one-year period. In all, they made sixty-two video recordings of eighteen children. The objective of the video recordings was not only to study patterns of communication in the classroom but also to observe how the educational program was organized.

Analysis of the video recordings showed that the way the children interacted in the school situation was congruent with the descriptions given by teachers, parents, and teacher assistants in the interviews. For the children in the general education classes, communication was based on speech. The teacher assistants tried to interpret what the teacher said into sign language, but the target child seldom looked continuously at the assistant, and therefore, it was difficult to assess what the child understood. From the way the children behaved and the questions they asked after the lesson, it was obvious that a lot of information had not been received. The children seldom made utterances in the classroom setting while the camera was on. They communicated with the teachers in spoken language, generally supported by nonverbal means or single signs in one-to-one settings. Some of the children signed to their assistants; others understood Swedish Sign Language to varying degrees, but were not observed using it. A lot of information that was communicated to the hearing children through short discussions with, or comments from, the teacher was seldom or never translated into sign language for the children with cochlear implants and therefore was not accessible to them.

In the classroom setting, the target child was often seated three to four meters from the teacher. Whether this spacing was an optimal hearing distance had never or seldom been discussed with the teachers. In several classes, the child had a good view of the teacher and the assistant but not of the other children because those children were seated beside or behind the child with a cochlear implant. Consequently, it was difficult for the deaf child to hear or see either what the other children said in the classroom or what answers those children gave to the teacher's questions. When the children with cochlear implants spoke, their difficulty articulating words and pronouncing consonants often made it difficult to understand what they had uttered. Their vocal tone was low and, in many cases, their vocabulary restricted. They had obvious problems taking part in a dialogue. Monologues more frequently occurred and could more easily be understood. Several of the children with cochlear implants often yawned and looked tired or disinterested when the whole class was gathered and the teacher was giving information or instructions. This reaction probably resulted because of their difficulty understanding what was said and their subsequent loss of interest and attention. When the child with a cochlear implant communicated with hearing peers, it was by a combination of not only nonverbal means and speech but also signs because some of the hearing children understood and could produce single signs.

In the special schools, the children with cochlear implants took part in the lessons in a way that differed significantly from the children in the general education classes. Because the class sizes were small (between six and twelve students in the special schools compared with eighteen to thirty students in the regular schools), it was difficult for them to be inattentive. Swedish Sign Language was used for instruction and communication, and the children appeared to have no difficulty understanding what the teachers and their peers signed. Some of the children in the special schools took part in sophisticated discussions about word meanings and could analyze language in a way that was not observed or registered among the children with cochlear implants in the regular classes.

The Children's Views on Using a Cochlear Implant

According to the UN Declaration of the Rights of the Child (UN 1989), issues concerning children should be dealt with from the child's own perspective. Young children, however, are seldom asked about their opinions on issues concerning their own lives. Previously, it has not been possible to ask many implanted children about their opinions and life experiences because they have been too young to respond. But because the first operations abroad were made in the late 1980s and early 1990s, the first generation of children with implants are now beginning to be old enough to express their opinion on wearing an implant. In a Norwegian study, eleven children who were ten- to nineteen-year-olds were interviewed about communicative strategies in interpersonal interaction (Christophersen 2001). Similar interviews were part of the Swedish psychosocial longitudinal study (Preisler, Tvingstedt, and Ahlström 2005).

In the Swedish psychosocial study, eleven of the oldest children were interviewed about their opinion on wearing an implant. Six of the children attended special schools for deaf students and five were in general education classes. The children were between the ages of eight and a half years and ten and a half years and had been wearing their implants between five and seven and a half years. Interviews with the children were conducted in their usual form of communication: (a) Swedish Sign Language with students in the special schools and (b) speech, with signs as support, with the children in regular settings.

It turned out that some of the children had memories from the time of the operation. They said that they experienced a strange sound when the processor was turned on. All but one of the eleven children used the implant daily. They said that it enabled them to perceive sounds in the environment, something they considered to be positive. Some of the children had experienced technical difficulties with the processor, for example, battery problems, wires that were too long and could be enervating, and processor breakdown. Most of the children had head-worn processors, which they thought were better than the early processors worn on a belt around the waist.

Most of the children reported experiencing difficulty taking part in conversations at home. The implant enabled them to perceive and understand simple statements, questions, or comments, but it did not give them access to more sophisticated discussion or advanced reasoning. The children's parents and teachers shared this opinion. The children in the special school considered speech to be difficult. Sign language was preferred, although several of the children in the special school were considered to have a good command of spoken Swedish. When asked what they could hear in general education classes, the children said that it was difficult for them to perceive what was said in class. The explanation was that the teachers and the other pupils were difficult to understand because their tone of voice was too weak or their way of speaking was slurred. The children with implants also found the sound level in the classroom disturbingly loud. The children's opinion about using the implant was in many ways similar to the opinion of their parents and teachers. They recognized advantages with the implant, but it did not enable them to fully participate in a hearing and speaking environment. The children identified their need for sign language, just as their parents and teachers had done. They said that peer interaction was best when the other children knew at least some sign language.

DISCUSSION

The researchers conducting the Swedish longitudinal study of psychosocial consequences for deaf children using cochlear implants have tried to shed light on the children's situation from the different perspectives of parents, teachers, and the children themselves. This method of triangulation has been one way of validating the research findings. The perspective of most of the team members of the two clinics where the implant operations were performed at the time the study began was that cochlear implantation was an option for deaf children to be able to perceive sounds and, hopefully, in the long term, to be able to speak and hear. Their knowledge of the consequences of deafness on a person's life, child development in general, and deaf children in particular was limited and in many cases nonexistent. These team members were the people who met with the parents of deaf children and were charged with the responsibility of providing information about the consequences of implantation on language development.

From the perspective of most of the parents in the study, the implant was regarded as a means of enabling the child to become bilingual in Swedish Sign Language and spoken Swedish. For most families in the study, sign language was already a natural means of communication before the operation (there were some exceptions; some postlingually deaf children received an implant shortly after becoming deaf as a result of meningitis). Two or three years after implantation, most parents found at least some of their hopes and expectations had been fulfilled. Their children could take part in simple spoken conversation in the home environment, although sign language was considered a necessity to understand and explain more complicated subjects. The situation was similar in the preschool and later in the school setting. Two parents said that they considered their child to be bilingual. These children had access to both languages: Swedish Sign Language in the special school during school hours and spoken Swedish in the hearing environment the rest of the time.

The teachers in the special schools regarded the children with cochlear implants as they would any other deaf child. They maintained that in the educational setting, sign language was necessary for the children to understand instructions and grasp more abstract reasoning. In the general educational classes, the teachers had no prior experience of deaf or hard of hearing children and, at first, were impressed by the children's way of adapting to the school situation. After a couple of years of experience having a child with a cochlear implant in their class, they became less enthusiastic about the classroom situation because the child with a cochlear implant had difficulty understanding and following the educational curriculum in spoken Swedish. The children provided a similar picture of their experience of the school situation. They were used to wearing the implant and found it useful in many circumstances. But to fully understand what was said at home and in the classroom setting, they needed sign language.

The question posed at the beginning of this chapter was whether deaf children's quality of life is enhanced with a cochlear implant. Because sign language has had a strong position in Sweden for the last thirty years, it is no understatement to maintain that the situation has radically changed within just a few years. When Swedish Sign Language was accepted as the first language of deaf children and when the goal of education was bilingualism, deaf children were given opportunities to acquire language spontaneously. The effect turned out to be very positive on the children's communicative, language, social, and cognitive development (Nordén et al. 1981; Preisler 1983; Heiling 1995; Preisler and Ahlström 1997).

These results are in accordance with the latest findings in developmental psychology that the roots of language are to be found in the early preverbal communication between parent and child where each shares the focus of attention in joyful and meaningful interaction. Oral language has long been regarded as a communication system that stands apart from the use of gestures and other nonverbal means of communication. However, recent research in linguistics and psycholinguistics regard the vocal and gestural systems as part of the same language system (McNeill 2000; Armstrong, Stokoe, and Wilcox 1995; Corballis 2002). The use of signs has long been considered a hinderance to the development of speech. However, studies now provide clear evidence that the use of gestures with hearing children is a transitional device en route to the use of two-word spoken utterances (Iverson, Capirci, and Caselli 1994; Capirci et al. 1996).

For the young deaf child, as for any child, the use of gestures is the most natural means of communication. A particularly significant finding in the psychosocial study of the preschool children with a cochlear implant was that the children with well-functioning speech also had good command of sign language (Preisler, Tvingstedt, and Ahlström 1999). This finding provides clear evidence that the use of signs can promote speech development. Another important prerequisite for language development is engagement in symbolic play in which children learn to handle symbols and representations of objects. Knowledge of how to communicate and play usually leads to positive peer interactions. Children need opportunities to communicate with others in a way that enables them to understand and be understood. In communication with others, concepts and meanings develop and new knowledge can be assimilated.

The results from the Swedish longitudinal study show that children with cochlear implants face considerable communicative obstacles in the home and classroom setting when communication is based only on speech. Their language skills remain inadequate for full functioning in a hearing environment. The presence of an adult who acts as mediator or interpreter in the classroom does not promote the development of friendships or normal peer relations. The children in such a context lack opportunities to discuss important matters with peers their own age. Studies of children's interaction with hearing peers show that the situation for children with implants closely resembles the experiences of hard of hearing children in settings with hearing peers (see, for example, Tvingstedt 1998; Antia and Kreimeyer 2003). The use of an implant does not resolve the difficulties in social interaction (Spencer and Marschark 2003). These results are confirmed in other studies (see Boyd, Knutson, and Dalstrom 2000). Thus, the results give cause for apprehension. As the children grow older, there will be greater demands made on their language and communication skills. Will these children manage to pass exams as well as to take part in higher education and in cultural and social activities where language plays a crucial role? These and many other questions remain unanswered.

In a study by Wald and Knutson (2000), deaf adolescents with and without implants were given the Deaf Identity Developmental Scale. Both groups tended to give the highest ratings to a "bicultural" identity; they wanted to be deaf but also part of the hearing society. This outcome is probably the case for most deaf people. Therefore, an important goal for the future is to enable deaf children with cochlear implants to construct such an identity. This goal requires that signed language must have as important a role in their lives as spoken language. Nine out of ten deaf children live in hearing families where they are exposed to speech daily. More attention must therefore be given to providing them with similar exposure to sign language if we are to enable them to develop a bicultural identity. By providing a truly bilingual context, the consequence will hopefully be a positive psychosocial development and better quality of life.

REFERENCES

Ahlström, M., A.-L. Tvingstedt, and G. Preisler. 1999. *Kommunikation och samspel i förskolemiljö* (Communication and interaction in the preschool setting). Pedagogisk-psykologiska Problem Report 665, Department of Educational and Psychological Research, School of Education, Malmö University, Malmö, Sweden (in Swedish).

Allen, M., T. Nikolopoulos, and G. O'Donoghue. 1998. Speech intelligibility in children after cochlear implantation. *American Journal of Otology* 19 (6):742–46.

Antia, S. D., and K. H. Kreimeyer. 2003. Peer interaction of deaf and hard of hearing children. In *Oxford handbook of deaf studies, language and education*, ed. P. E. Spencer and M. Marschark, 164–76. Oxford: Oxford University Press.

Archbold,S., M. Lutman, S. Gregory, C. O'Neill, and T. Nikolopoulos. 2002. Parents and their deaf child: Their perceptions three years after cochlear implantation. *Deafness and Educational International* 4 (1):12–40.

Armstrong, D. F., W. C. Stokoe, and S. E. Wilcox. 1995. *Gesture and the nature of language*. Cambridge: Cambridge University Press.

Barnes, S., M. Gutfreund, D. Satterly, and G. Wells. 1983. Characteristics of adult speech which predict children's language development. *Journal of Child Language* 10: 65–84.

Blamey, P. J., J. Sarant, L. Paatsch, J. Barry, C. Bow, R. Wales, M. Wright, C. Psarros, K. Rattigan, and R. Tooher. 2001. Relationships among speech perception, production, language, hearing loss, and age in children with impaired hearing. *Journal of Speech, Language and Hearing Research* 44: 264–85.

Blume, S. 2002. Technology, medicine, and the quality of life. In *Barn och unge med cochlea implantat. Utvikling och livskvalitet. Rapport fra nordisk konferense in Oslo 21–23 November 2001 (Children and adolescents with cochlear implants. Development and quality of life. Report from a Nordic Conference in Oslo, November 21–23, 2001)*, ed. E. Simonsen, U. Jochumsen, and A.-E., Kristoffersen, 69–86. Skådalen Publication Series 14. Oslo, Norway: Skådalen Resource Center.

Boyd, R., J. Knutson, and A. Dalstrom. 2000. Social interaction of pediatric cochlear implant recipients with age-matched peers. *Annals of Otology, Rhinology and Laryngology* 109 (Suppl. 185):105–9.

Capirci, O., J. M. Iverson, E. Pizzuto, and V. Volterra. 1996. Gestures and words during the transition to two-word speech. *Journal of Child Language* 23: 645–73.

Christophersen, A. B. 2001. *Barn og unge med cochleaimplantat. Hvordan opplever de sin kommunikasjonssituation. (Children and adolescents with cochlear implants: How they experience their own communicative situation)*. Skådalen Publication Series 11. Oslo, Norway: Skådalen Resource Center.

Corballis, M. C. 2002. *From hand to mouth: The origins of language*. Princeton, N.J.: Princeton University Press.

Fogel, A. 1993. *Developing through relationships. Origins of communication, self, and culture*. New York: Harvester Wheatsheaf.

Geers, A., and J. Moog. 1994. Effectiveness of cochlear implant and tactile aids for deaf children: The sensory aids study at Central Institute for the Deaf [Monograph]. *The Volta Review* 96 (5):97–108.

Gregory, S. 2002. Issues in assessing the quality of life of deaf children and their families. In *Barn och unge med cochlea implantat. Utvikling och livskvalitet. Rapport fra nordisk konferense in Oslo 21–23 November 2001 (Children and adolescents with cochlear implants. Development and quality of life. Report from a Nordic Conference in Oslo, November 21–23, 2001)*, ed. E. Simonsen, U. Jochumsen, and A.-E. Kristoffersen, 59–68. Skådalen Publication Series 14. Oslo, Norway: Skådalen Resource Center.

Heiling, K. 1995. *The development of deaf children: Academic achievement levels and social processes*. Hamburg: Signum.

Hoff-Ginsberg, E., and M. Schatz. 1982. Linguistic input and the child's acquisition of language. *Psychological Bulletin* 92: 3–26.

Iverson, J. M., O. Capirci, and M. C. Caselli. 1994. From communication to language in two modalities. *Cognitive Development* 9: 23–43.

Jorup, B., and G. Preisler. 2001. *Lekens plats i förskolan för barn med cochlea implantat. Analys av lekobservationer i olika pedagogiska miljöer (Play in the preschool setting for children with cochlear implants. Analysis of play observations in different educational settings)*. Report 112, Department of Psychology, Stockholm University, Sweden (in Swedish).

Kluwin, T. N., and D. A. Stewart. 2000. Cochlear implants for young children: A preliminary description of the parental decision, process and outcomes. *American Annals of the Deaf* 145 (1):22–32.

Kugiumutzakis, G. 1998. Neonatal imitation in the intersubjective companion in space. In *Intersubjective communication and emotion in early ontogeny*, ed. S. Bråten, 63–88. Cambridge: Cambridge University Press.

MacDonald, J. D., and J. Y. Carroll. 1994. Adult communication styles: The missing link to early language intervention. *Infant-Toddler Intervention* 4 (3):145–60.

Martin, D., and Y. Bat-Chava. 2003. Negotiating deaf-hearing friendships: Coping strategies of deaf boys and girls in mainstream schools. *Child, Care Health and Development* 29 (6):511–21.

McNeill, D. 2000. *Language and gesture*. Cambridge: Cambridge University Press.

Meyer, T., M. Svirsky, K. Kirk, and R. Miyamoto. 1998. Improvements in speech perception by children with profound prelingual hearing loss: Effects of device, communication mode and chronological age. *Journal of Speech, Language, and Hearing Research* 41 (4):846–58.

Miyamoto, R., A. Robbins, M. J. Osberger, S. Todd, I. Allyson, M. Riley, and K. Kirk. 1995. Comparison of multichannel tactile aids and multichannel cochlear implants in children with profound hearing impairments. *American Journal of Otology* 16 (1):8–13.

Moseley, M. J. 1990. Mother-child interaction with preschool language-delayed children: Structuring conversations. *Journal of Communication Disorders* 23 (3):187–203.

Nadel, J., C. Guérini, A. Pezé, and C. Rivet. 1999. The evolving nature of imitation as a format for communication. In *Imitation in infancy*, ed. J. Nadel and G. Butterworth, 209–34. Cambridge: Cambridge University Press.

Nordén, K., G. Preisler, K. Heiling, E. Hülphers, and A.-L. Tvingstedt. 1981. Learning processes and personality development in deaf children. *International Journal of Rehabilitation Research* 4 (3):393–95.

O'Neill, C., S. M. Archbold, G. M. O'Donoghue, D. A. McAlister, and T. P. Nikolopoulos. 2001. Indirect costs, cost-utility variations and the funding of paediatric cochlear implantation. *International Journal of Pediatric Otorhinolaryngology* 58 (1):53–57.

Preisler, G. 1983. Deaf children in communication. Ph.D. diss., Department of Psychology, Stockholm University.

———. 2001. *Cochlear implants in deaf children*. Report for the Committee on the Rehabilitation and Integration of People with Disabilities. Strasbourg: Council of Europe Publishing.

Preisler, G., and M. Ahlström. 1997. Sign language for hard of hearing children: A hindrance or a benefit for their development? *European Journal of Psychology of Education.* 12 (4):465–77.

Preisler, G., M. Ahlström, and A.-L. Tvingstedt. 1997. The development of communication and language in deaf preschool children with cochlear implants. *International Journal of Pediatric Otorhinolaryngology* 41: 263–72.

Preisler, G., A.-L. Tvingstedt, and M. Ahlström. 1999. *Mötet mellan föräldrar och CI-team samt mötet mellan föreskolepersonal och CI-team. (The meeting between parents, and CI-team and preschool staff and implant team).* Pedagogisk-psykologiska Problem Report 663, Department of Educational and Psychological Research, School of Education, Malmö University, Sweden (in Swedish).

———. 2002. A psycho-social follow-up study of deaf preschool children using cochlear implants. *Child: Care, Health and Development* 28 (5):403–18.

———. 2003. *Skolsituationen för barn med CI—Ur föräldrars, lärares och assistenters perspektiv (The school situation of children with CI—From the perspective of parents, teachers and personal assistants).* Report 116, Department of Psychology, Stockholm University, Sweden (in Swedish).

———. 2005. Interviews with children with cochlear implants. *American Annals of the Deaf.*

———. Forthcoming. Video observations of school children with cochlear implants in regular classes and in special schools for the deaf and hard of hearing.

Rizzolatti, G., and M. A. Arbib. 1998. Language within our grasp. *Trends in the Neurosciences* 21: 188–94.

Spencer, P. E., and M. Marschark. 2003. Cochlear implants: Issues and implications. In *Oxford handbook of deaf studies, language and education,* ed. P. E. Spencer and M. Marschark, 434–48. Oxford: Oxford University Press.

Stern, D. 2000. *The interpersonal world of the infant. A view from psychoanalysis and developmental psychology.* New York: Basic Books. (Orig. pub. 1985.)

Svirsky, M., A. K. Robbins, K. I. Kirk, D. B. Pisoni, and R. T. Miyamoto. 2000. Language development in profoundly deaf children with cochlear implants. *Psychological Science* 11 (2):153–58.

Swedish National Board of Health and Welfare. 2000. *Vårdprogram för barn med cochlea implantat (Directions for habilitation of children with cochlear implants).* Report 2000:06, Swedish National Board of Health and Welfare, Stockholm.

Trevarthen, C. 2004. How infants learn how to mean. In *A learning zone of one's own,* M. Tokoro and L. Steels, 37–70. Amsterdam: IOS Press.

Tronick, E. Z. 1998. Dyadically expanded states of consciousness and the process of therapeutic change. *Infant Mental Health Journal* 19 (3):290–99.

Tvingstedt, A.-L. 1998. Classroom interaction and the social situation of hard-of-hearing pupils in regular classes. In *Proceedings of the 18th International Congress on Education of the Deaf—1995. Tel-Aviv, Israel,* ed. A. Weisel, 406–11. Tel Aviv: Ramot Publications, Tel Aviv University. (ERIC Document Reproduction Service ED 392188)

Tvingstedt, A.-L., G. Preisler, and M. Ahlström. 1999. *Cochlea implantat på barn: En psykosocial uppföljningsstudie. Kommunikation och samspel i familjen (Cochlear implants in children: A psychosocial follow-up study. Communication and interaction in the family).* Pedagogisk-psykologiska Problem Report 664, Department of Educational and Psychological Research, School of Education, Malmö University, Malmö, Sweden (in Swedish).

———. 2000. Communication with deaf pre-school children using cochlear implants. Paper presented at the 19th International Congress on Education of the Deaf, ICED 2000, July 9–13, Sydney, Australia.

———. 2001. Pre-school children with cochlear implants: A psycho social follow up study. Paper presented at the Sign Language as a Guide to Dutch conference, November 15–16, Groningen, Netherlands.

———. 2003. *Skolplacering av barn med cochlea implantat (School placement of children with cochlear implants)*. Report 115, Department of Psychology, Stockholm University (in Swedish).

United Nations (UN). 1989. *Declaration of the rights of the child.* http://www.unhchr.ch/html/menu3/b/k2crc/htm.

Wald, R., and J. Knutson. 2000. Deaf cultural identity of adolescents with and without cochlear implants. *Annals of Otology, Rhinology and Laryngology* 109 (Suppl 185):87–89.

7

COCHLEAR-IMPLANTED CHILDREN IN SWEDEN'S BILINGUAL SCHOOLS

Kristina Svartholm

A growing number of deaf children with cochlear implants are entering Swedish schools for deaf students. Although many parents are choosing a cochlear implant for their deaf children, Swedish parents also call for Swedish Sign Language to be used in these schools. This chapter sets out the dilemma that the special schools face. The central question considered here is whether it is possible for one and the same school to offer a language setting that will suit *all* deaf children, with or without a cochlear implant, or will one of these two groups of children be the loser. The knowledge gained from more than two decades of sign language research and bilingual educational practices in Sweden is vital for our understanding of how to best cope with the new situation created by the increase in childhood implantation.

After some years of decline in school enrollment in schools for deaf and hard of hearing students in Sweden,[1] a new trend is clearly discernible. There are slightly more children now enrolled in schools for deaf students than in the previous three to five years. One explanation put forward by the National Agency for Special Schools for the Deaf and Hard of Hearing (Specialskolemyndigheten; SPM) is that parents of children with cochlear implants seem to be choosing schools with a signing setting to a larger extent than before. These parents want their children to develop bilingualism in Swedish (spoken and written) and Swedish Sign Language (see Preisler this volume). Another explanation is that the special schools are now seeing a number of older students who have a greater need for sign language than first expected when their parents chose local school placement among hearing children (SPM 2004).

This situation clearly puts new demands on the schools for deaf students. There is a steadily growing group of children with cochlear implants whose parents expect not only bilingualism, as traditionally provided by the schools, but also speech training and use of spoken language. This expectation presupposes a new pedagogical approach that is somewhat different from the way schools for deaf students in Sweden have worked over the past twenty to twenty-five years. The situation is further complicated by Sweden's small population. The number of children born deaf or with a hearing impairment (severe enough to require the use of hearing aids) is approximately 200 annually. Of this number, approximately fifty to sixty deaf and hard of hearing children are enrolled at each grade level in special schools for deaf students around Sweden.[2]

Despite the growing number of children with implants who are attending schools for deaf students in Sweden, the vast majority of children enrolled in these schools are deaf students without implants. Even if this group successively becomes smaller because of the large number of implant operations being conducted in Sweden, there will always be those who remain deaf and are not implanted for one reason or another. These children must be guaranteed continuing access to bilingual education to develop Swedish Sign Language and written Swedish language proficiency, the kind of bilingual program that has been so successful in developing these skills in the past. It is a delicate task for the schools to combine this kind of bilingual program with an education for deaf children with implants for whom speech and hearing are important. Another group, older children who need remedial teaching, require a bilingual program that targets not only language development but also development of knowledge that has been missed earlier in their schooling. Moreover, it can be expected that many of these children will need extra support to restore their self-esteem and to establish a strong identity after having "failed" among hearing children in regular schools.

One option to accommodate the differing needs of implanted and non-implanted children would be to create two separate and different types of schools, but ones in which sign language holds a prominent position. This effort would be rather difficult to carry out. Dividing the population in this way would mean that the number of children in each type of school would probably be so small that it would be difficult to maintain a satisfactory signing environment. Besides, this kind of accommodation is not what parents want when they choose a special school for their child. Instead, developmental work must take place to make the bilingual schools for deaf students in Sweden work as well for children with implants as for those without.

BILINGUAL EDUCATION IN THE SPECIAL SCHOOL

The following section gives a short description of the development of bilingual education within special schools for the deaf and hard of hearing in Sweden. It begins with the situation soon after 1981, when Swedish Sign Language was first recognized as the language of deaf people in Sweden, and outlines the main ideas behind the curricula work that has been carried out since then.

The First Important Steps

Contrary to the apparent belief of many people around the world, speech has never been banned or excluded from Swedish schools for the deaf. The 1983 Special School Curriculum document (LGr 80 Spec 1983), which supplemented the 1980 Compulsory School Curriculum (LGr 80 1980), stated that deaf children should strive toward bilingualism, with Swedish Sign Language as their first language and Swedish as their second language (that is, to be able to read and write Swedish). It also directed that students with residual hearing (such that they could profit from instruction through spoken language if assisted by technical devices) should be taught in groups of their own whenever possible. Furthermore, it identified the need for careful consideration about whether deaf students should also use spoken language and not solely sign language. In the year 2004 22 percent of the deaf and hearing impaired children in Swedish schools for deaf students were instructed, to some degree, in speech (SPM 2004a).

In the bilingual program for deaf students, the functional differentiation of the two languages, Swedish Sign Language and Swedish, is emphasized. Sign language is described as the primary tool for acquiring knowledge and the language used in face-to-face interaction with others. Swedish primarily fulfills the functions of written language, but speechreading and speech are also important parts of the school curriculum (see Svartholm 1993 for a discussion of the use of the two languages as a form of *diglossia*). The Swedish National Association for the Deaf (SDR 1996, 28) described the role of speech in deaf education as enabling a deaf person to "use speech when necessary, not to communicate in spoken language."

The years following the introduction of the Special School Curriculum can be best characterized as a period of intense pioneer work—in research, in teaching, and in developmental work of different kinds (such as resource development with teachers, discussions of linguistic devices, pedagogical approaches, and so on). Special focus was put on the needs of young deaf children and their parents; in early intervention programs, hearing parents were encouraged to learn sign language and were offered courses in this language without charge. Their children were provided with day-care activities in which Swedish Sign Language was used throughout the day by other deaf children and adults, deaf and hearing. Consequently, more and more deaf children entered school with the same expectations as hearing children and with similar, seemingly age-appropriate social, cognitive, and linguistic development (Mahshie 1995).

In coping with this new situation, all teachers for deaf students underwent in-service training in Swedish Sign Language. Many of them were also trained to teach the new school subject Swedish as a second language for the deaf. The focus was on literacy development, contrasting and comparing written Swedish with Swedish Sign Language. The training programs extended over several years and concurrently with the development of teaching materials and resources for working bilingually with deaf students in the schools. The growing number of teachers who were themselves deaf was a very important part of the development of bilingual education programs in Sweden. These teachers were qualified by teacher training institutions (colleges and universities), some of them specializing in Swedish Sign Language and Swedish as a second language for the deaf. The fact that speech and speech training had to make way for these additional subjects and new approaches to deaf education is no surprise. The schools chose different ways of offering speech training, depending on students' preferences. The central view was that speech training should be voluntary and individualized, even though some training could be carried out in small groups. The focus, however, was on sign language and written language as the basis for deaf bilingualism.

Raising the Standards

The model of bilingual education in Sweden has changed the attitudes toward deaf children. Teachers found their pupils to be fully competent with the same capacity for learning as hearing children. Thus, a new perspective on deaf children and their prospects gradually arose. This development undoubtedly resulted from the strong position assigned to Swedish Sign Language as the primary language for deaf children. This perspective was clearly reflected in a new national curriculum for the compulsory school system, including special schools (LPO 94 1994). Until then, schools were obliged to ensure deaf students' development *toward* bilingualism (LGr 80 Spec 1983). Now, the goal of bilingualism was expressed in a more definite way:

> Schools for pupils with impaired hearing/vision and speech disabilities are responsible for ensuring that all pupils, who are deaf or have impaired hearing, on completing school are bilingual, i.e., can read sign language and Swedish as well as express thoughts and ideas in both sign language and writing, [can] can communicate in writing in English. (LPO 94 1994, 19)

The curriculum was followed by new syllabi, the same as those for hearing pupils except for the language-specific subjects Swedish Sign Language, Swedish as a second language for deaf students, and music (which became "movement and drama" for deaf students). The curriculum goals, general and subject-specific, were consistent for deaf and hearing students across all schools.

The necessity for all deaf and hard of hearing pupils to have some general knowledge about the workings of speech was explicitly noted in the curriculum (Skolverket 1996), as was the need for knowledge about the use of spoken language, including its use by sign language interpreters. Individually adapted speech training was still offered (to varying degrees in different schools) according to what parents and pupils requested.

A Special School, Available for All

Soon after the 1996 syllabi were decided, a public committee for disabled students in school, known as FUNKIS (*Funktionshindrade elever i skolan*), began its work. The committee's main task was to clarify whether the responsibility for education of students with disabilities should remain with the national government or be transferred to local school authorities. The latter alternative would open the possibility for decisions about the role and use of sign language in schools for deaf students to be made at the local level.

The committee's final report especially attended to children with cochlear implants (FUNKIS 1998). The report stated that the children's capacity to hear must be assessed individually; some had achieved the prerequisites for developing spoken Swedish, and some had not. Furthermore, it was stated that pupils with cochlear implants should be given the opportunity to develop and consolidate their sign language and spoken Swedish. The committee reported that three out of the (then) five special schools instructed some students in groups, using spoken Swedish with technical aids, and some students in classes that used Swedish Sign Language the language of instruction (FUNKIS 1998). One of the committee's recommendations was to extend this opportunity to choose between languages (Swedish Sign Language or spoken Swedish) to all five special schools.

The government used this report to draft a bill later passed by the Swedish Parliament (Proposition 1998/99, 105) that accentuated the need for sign language among the deaf, the deaf-blind, and some hard of hearing children. The bill explicitly stated that the special schools for deaf and hard of hearing students were obliged to "offer a sign language environment in which everyone, as much as possible, communicates in signs" (my translation). The bill also stressed that such an environment could not be provided by integrating individuals or small groups of deaf students who needed sign language into regular schools. The government remained responsible to ensure a sign language environment within the special schools for deaf and hard of hearing students. Further, the bill made explicit reference to the United Nations *Standard Rules on the Equalization of Opportunities for Persons with Disabilities* (UN 1993), which states the need for special schools and access to instruction in sign language for deaf students.

Soon after 1996, work on revising the syllabi for schools for deaf students began again. The group charged with this task thoroughly discussed whether two different syllabi were needed: one for deaf children, the other for hard of hearing children and children with cochlear implants. Group members decided that there would be only one syllabus, written so that "it gives the opportunity and responsibility for the schools to meet every child considering his or her specific needs and qualifications" (Henning 2003, 35). Henning, who actively participated in this work, pointed out that schools for deaf students must provide "a highly qualified sign language environment with the aim of bilingualism" (2003, 35) but that each school had the freedom to choose teaching methods and goals for individual pupils.

In the guidelines for special schools, the two languages—Swedish Sign Language and Swedish—are now considered more or less in unity. An introductory section of the syllabus describes the interdependence of these two languages for personal development and learning. Signing, speaking, reading, and writing are core areas that are highlighted; the pupils should be given the opportunity to use and develop their skills as individuals, as appropriate to their individual abilities.

Thus, the curriculum and its syllabi express the intentions of the special school to be available to all, to be flexible, and to account for everyone's needs. The questions now are How well do children with cochlear implants fit into this school system? Are there special adaptations that should be made to fulfill their individual needs? Or are special adaptations needed to fulfill the needs of those deaf children without implants who may well become a minority within this new, flexible special school system?

WHICH LANGUAGE—AND WHEN?

From research reported by Preisler and others (see this volume) we know that the parents of the first generation of children with cochlear implants in Sweden have expressed their desire for more speech training for their children in the schools for deaf students. At the same time, they expressed satisfaction with the educational level achieved through the use of sign language in these schools. Their request for more speech indicated that they sought something beyond the usual academic achievement being attained by deaf students.

Offering speech training of the conventional kind, in more or less individual settings, generally did not satisfy the parents. Successive discussions with the schools included demands for spoken language use in the classroom. Adopting the recommendations of the FUNKIS committee, the SPM presented the following guidelines for special schools:

These special schools offer students

a. Instruction in Sign Language or speech, with the possibility of choosing different instructional languages for different subjects and even changing the choice during the course of schooling
b. An individual development plan
c. Training in sound and speech stimulation and speech training tailored to individual needs and choices
d. Teachers who are deaf, hard-of-hearing and hearing. (SPM 2004b)

Accordingly, children with cochlear implants are now offered instruction through spoken language as an alternative to sign language, depending on their parents' wishes. Consequently, some, if not all, of their scholastic attainment should be gained through speech.

Unfortunately, there is still very little knowledge about how the use of spoken language in the teaching situation works in practice with these children. Furthermore, we do not know yet what their achievements will be and whether they will reach an appropriate educational level. It is also unknown whether they will reach a satisfactory level of bilingualism in line with the achievements of most deaf children in Sweden today. Will speech really provide these children with an optimal learning environment? How can speech interplay with sign language so the goal of bilingualism can be attained for children with cochlear implants?

USE OF SPEECH IN CLASS

Preisler (see this volume) reports problems for children with cochlear implants who participate in general educational classes. In particular, difficulties arise with participation in oral dialogue. One premise, important when speech is to be used as the language of instruction, is that many children with cochlear implants cannot be expected to follow spoken language in full, especially when it is used within a group. Situations in which there is more than one interlocutor may be strenuous for many implant recipients, even if the group is small and the atmosphere friendly.

The difficulty for people with impaired hearing in oral group discussions is well known. This situation is particularly difficult when there are more than three or four participants. The exact number of participants with which a person with impaired hearing can cope may vary because of the physical setting and the individual's capacity for hearing (Ahlström and Svartholm 1998). This knowledge and its implications should be considered carefully before any decisions are made about using speech as the language of instruction for groups of children with impaired hearing. Is the size of the instructional group adapted to suit each child's ability so she or he can participate efficiently? If not, some students will remain outside the group and be excluded from the language used within it.

Extra consideration must be given to yet another fact. Children are in the process of developing language skills, and their respective linguistic levels may vary considerably. Therefore, it may be that what causes problems is not only the group interaction but also the language used for the interaction. If the child has difficulty not only following what is going on in the group but also understanding the language used by others, then the learning situation is less favorable. If the children participating also have difficulty in speech production, articulation, and pronunciation, then they will distort the speech sounds and make it more difficult for the other children in the group to get the message by ear. This possibility, of course, makes the situation even less effective.

Some of the problems connected to the use of speech in situations of this kind could probably be overcome, at least to some extent. One approach is to pay extra attention to the communicative situation as such. A well-developed responsibility for group communication (obedience to rather strict rules for turn taking) has been identified among sign language users (see Svartholm, Andersson, and Lindahl 1993 for their description of a class of twenty-three deaf students in their last grade in school). Students in the study were conscious of the need for eye contact with the whole group when signing in class. They distinctly showed when they wanted to join the discussion, motioning to the teacher or student in charge of the discussion. They were also careful about getting into a position in the classroom where they were visible to everyone before making a contribution. Thus, the discussions ran smoothly and were accessible to everyone in the room.

A similar consciousness about the needs of the group could well be expected from children with a hearing impairment who use speech, particularly if they are trained with relevant strategies. Using spoken language with small groups of children who show consideration for one another and adopt disciplined turn taking within the group may well offer a very positive oral setting for deaf children. But, as previously pointed out, there are problems connected to the fact that spoken language is not fully accessible to children with impaired hearing. Students will have problems, to a greater or lesser degree, perceiving the message. For this reason, some will remain as outsiders. A recommendation to teachers responsible for groups of this kind would be to pay extra attention to the need for discussion and free conversation among the children in the group. It has to be kept in mind that if students' participation in group discussions is limited, in all likelihood, so too will be their achievements.

There is one more important question to consider carefully. Will a communicative setting provided by the use of only speech promote complex language use among children with cochlear implants? The speech used by a group of children with impaired hearing may not provide opportunities to use language for more advanced functions such as talking about abstract matters, arguing, testing hypotheses, persuading, generalizing, drawing conclusions, and so on. The importance of children actively negotiating meaning with others at a more advanced level, whether they are first or second language learners, is incontestable. Such discussions promote not only language development but also higher cognitive functioning in the child. It is the kind of interpersonal communication that

Cummins (1996) describes as cognitively demanding and context-embedded, an essential aspect of academic language proficiency. Communicative proficiency of this type is the basis for other academic achievement. It would be unreasonable to expect learners to develop literacy for academic purposes without first securing opportunities to use language of this kind in interpersonal, face-to-face settings; it would be equally unreasonable if reading and writing were taught as contextualized skills.

Again, it must be questioned whether speech provides an optimal learning situation for these children. To develop new knowledge as well as the vocabulary and language structures connected to it, children need language to be used in meaningful contexts. For children who have difficulty fully comprehending spoken language, the introduction of new information by speech alone inappropriately risks that the acquisition of knowledge will be hampered.

SIGN SUPPORTED SPEECH IN CLASS?

An alternative to the speech-only classes for children with cochlear implants proposed by many parents today in Sweden is the use of sign-supported speech, known as *Tecken Som Stöd* (TSS). TSS is used with hard of hearing children in preschool activities and at school as well as among deafened or hard of hearing adults. However, although sign-supported speech is used by hard of hearing people in many everyday situations, very often their preference is for Swedish Sign Language to be used as a functional complement to spoken Swedish (Ahlström and Svartholm 1998).

The importance of native sign language was first recognized in Sweden in the early 1980s; however, Swedes do have experience using sign-supported speech in schools for deaf students for a period before that. Since its abandonment in the late 1970s, a return to TSS as a communicative approach to instruction has seldom been considered by educators. Nevertheless, given parents requests for TSS with children who have implants, it is important to look again at this approach. Is sign-supported speech an efficient way to promote children's language development? What do we know about it from a linguistic point of view?

As in many other countries, the simultaneous use of speech and signs was introduced in deaf education in Sweden in the late 1960s. The main characteristic of this approach, known as Signed Swedish, was that one word was supposed to correspond to one sign, and the order of signs was supposed to follow the word order of the spoken language. Signed Swedish was expected to enhance language learning among deaf people, that is, learning the language of the wider society (Swedish). These expectations, however, were not fulfilled. The approach seemed to work fairly well with young children to begin with, but as the children grew older, their linguistic development seemed to cease. Gradually, when knowledge from sign language research deepened, it became clear why this way of speaking and signing was inefficient as a tool for developing language.

The main explanation of the failure of constructed sign systems has to do with the production and perception of spoken language and sign language. Native sign languages are produced in ways that allow for a significantly higher degree of simultaneously produced linguistic information than is possible in spoken language (Bergman 1979, 1982). A well-known fact today is that native sign language uses nonmanual means (such as facial expression, mouth movements, direction of gaze, and so on) simultaneously with manual signs. Furthermore, native sign languages have spatial rather than temporal organization. The three-dimensional space in front of the signer is used in the language structure itself (Bergman 1990; Engberg-Pedersen 1993; see also Liddell 2003 for a thorough analysis of spatial uses of signs connected to mental space theory). The manifestation of this organization can be described to a large extent as following the principle of simultaneity, which is well suited to how the eye receives information (Bellugi 1980).

When signs are produced together with spoken words, following the word order of the spoken language, another principle takes over: temporal organization. That is, the dominant organization of spoken language applies, and one sign or one word follows another in time. The principle of temporal organization is highly suited to how the ear receives information, but less suited for the eye. Of crucial importance is that the linguistic information conveyed by the signs when produced in this way becomes reduced and fragmented, and the grammar becomes distorted.

The inadequate information conveyed through simultaneous communication becomes evident when we consider what is normally expressed by the prosodic elements of speech. This information, including intonation or stress, is not visually represented when using signs simultaneously with speech and must therefore be filled in by the receiver. Supplementing this information places great demands on the receiver and relies on his or her ability to do so; a high proficiency in the spoken language is required to do this supplementing efficiently and accurately. If the message is short and simple, then the demands on the receiver are not excessive. If the message is also bound to the immediate context, to the "here and now," it is easier to understand. This kind of communication is the way adults talk to young children and, presumably, why signing and speaking simultaneously initially seemed to function well with young deaf children (Ahlgren 1984).

Although the signs used in simultaneous communication with young deaf children were easily comprehensible for the most part, what the children saw was signs following one another with no grammatical links between them. The children could produce signs in an order that seemed to follow the Swedish word order in short, simple sentences, probably best described as a form of linguistic adjustment to a less fluent signer. The mouth movements used by the child together with the signs were taken as evidence of the child's knowledge of Swedish. However, to the child, the mouth movements did not represent Swedish words at all. Instead, for every single sign, the deaf child had to learn the corresponding Swedish word, both in speech and in writing.

The use of sign and speech may make it easier to speechread spoken language for the person who already knows the language. However, using that approach with deaf children with the intention of making linguistic information visually available for language learning cannot be justified linguistically. Instead, the model for bilingual teaching that has been developed over the years seems to better fulfill the goals of deaf education, including the development of literacy.

It is difficult to advocate the use of sign-supported speech for hearing impaired children if its use is supposed to make it easier for them to learn spoken language. Sign-supported speech may help the child develop speechreading skills, and it may help in understanding simple messages. However, expecting the child to learn new words and concepts from speech with accompanying signs seems a rather uncertain way to go. Here, it would be wise to listen to what is often asserted by hard of hearing young people and adults, namely, that their learning of new vocabulary in Swedish is largely connected to *reading* the language, not encountering new words in speech (Ahlström and Svartholm 1998).

When parents seek bilingualism for their child, it should be remembered that sign language is not learned from presenting signs simultaneously with speech. It is often reported that adults—including teachers who work with young deaf and hard of hearing children and who use short, simple sentences with them—have problems consistently representing words by signs (for example, see Hjulstad, Kristoffersen, and Simonsen 2002). As a result, the visually dependent child gets unsystematic and uneven linguistic input from sign-supported speech. In all likelihood, the signs will not be used consistently enough and in sufficient correspondence with native sign language for the child to develop a satisfactory lexical knowledge in Swedish, not to mention grammar skills in this language.

Sign Language and Bilingualism

As pointed out earlier, many parents of children with cochlear implants seem to be well aware of the need for their children to be bilingual. They realize that their child will need sign language not only during school but also later in life. Some parents seem to consider sign language as more or less a "life jacket" for their child: if anything happens to the implant later on, the child may become totally deaf and dependent on signing.

The parents interviewed in Preisler and colleagues' study (see Preisler this volume) maintained the importance of sign language when explaining complicated, abstract, especially important information or new concepts to their children. But how can this level of language use be attained by children with implants? Is it sufficient to place the child in a special school for him or her to encounter sign language outside class, during breaks, and in physical activities conducted with other deaf children?

When parents make a claim for speech instead of sign language as the language of instruction for their children, they apparently take a risk on the bilingual development of their child, something that many of them seem quite unaware of. If children do not encounter sign language used in connection to different areas of the curriculum, in different situations, by different people, for different purposes, then they may eventually experience undesired gaps in their vocabulary and in their command of different linguistic domains. The concept of linguistic domains was originally presented by Fishman in two now classic articles about speech situations of different kinds (Fishman 1965, 1972). His work is valuable not least for identifying different uses of language that language learners encounter and the uses of language expected from them. These domains can be described as, for example, use of language in everyday conversation within the family, use of language for social purposes with friends in and outside school, use of language in formal situations with strangers, and so on. The concept of linguistic domains can be further widened to include the vocabulary used within different situations.

At home and with friends, basic, everyday vocabulary is used; in formal situations and those connected to academic study and the professions, the vocabulary is of a more complex kind, generally speaking. This advanced vocabulary is supposed to develop largely during the school years.

But what can be expected to happen when a school child with impaired hearing encounters sign language only in basic, everyday situations, with friends inside and outside school? What will the restrictions be for language development? The negative consequences might be more profound than first expected, not least because the child may already be lagging behind in spoken language development and may be encountering speech that is, by necessity (as discussed earlier), simplified. If, for instance, reasoning connected to scientific phenomena and terminology is lacking in the language used with the child, whether spoken or signed, then no one could expect the corresponding conceptualization to take place. Because such conceptualization can be seen as a deeper understanding of everyday concepts, its underdevelopment may result in not only a vocabulary gap but also a lack of understanding of the conceptual networks that vocabulary represents.

Bilingualism involves more than sign language proficiency. Of course the goal in deaf education is also to provide students with linguistic input from, and experience with, the language of the wider society. It is a delicate task for the special school to find the right balance when fulfilling students' need to use speech with one or more interlocutors in different situations and for different purposes, without taking too much time from subject instruction. A carefully designed bilingual program in which sign language is used as the language of instruction must also highlight the role of written language.

A great challenge for bilingual special schools in Sweden is to scrutinize its experience of teaching literacy through native sign language to deaf children and adapting this methodology to best suit the needs of children with cochlear implants. It may be that the development of reading and writing skills among deaf children with implants, like deaf children without implants, is best done through vision. Alternatively, the use of both vision and previously developed spoken language skills may better assist these students. Much research and developmental work is needed. What is certain is that reading and writing will be of utmost importance for these children to continue to develop skills in Swedish, irrespective of how well they can use their implants for hearing.

CONCLUDING REMARKS

By providing opportunities for rich and profound sign language development in and outside the school, children with cochlear implants, and those with impaired hearing in general, will be better prepared for life after school. They will be able to use sign language interpreters when it is important that information be received accurately or when they are in group situations such as seminars and meetings. Sign language interpreters will likely make higher education accessible to many (or perhaps most) deaf and hearing impaired students. The importance of native sign language for these students is evidenced by the growing number of both hard of hearing and deaf students who are enrolled in higher education in Sweden and who use sign language interpreters. A person with impaired hearing is often excluded from group discussions; the ideal kinds of groups mentioned earlier in this chapter, in which participants adapt to one another's hearing impairment and the communicative needs connected to it, are not what the hearing impaired child will meet outside the school setting. In the less-than-ideal situations, interpreting will make participation possible. The strenuous task of listening—and the accompanying feelings of insecurity reported by many hard of hearing people—is overcome by the use of interpreters. There is no reason to believe that the situation for the current population of children with cochlear implants will be very different when they leave school.

Bilingual education for children with cochlear implants will result, in all likelihood, in better opportunities later in life. Mastering not only sign language but also the language of the broader society will make it possible for them to make their own life choices. Consideration of the linguistic needs of these children should be made with their lifelong prospects in mind.

Finally, the importance of an ethical standpoint in discussions and decision making about language use for deaf and hearing impaired students in special schools needs to be emphasized: Communication must be accessible and available to everyone. Speech may well be used in the classroom with children with cochlear implants if *all* the children manage to follow it. Outside the classroom, where deaf and hearing impaired children will meet, it is vital that sign language is used by everyone, both children and adults. If this ethical standpoint is strictly adhered to, then no children in the special schools for deaf students, with or without implants, will become losers.

NOTES

1. The decline in school enrollment, generally speaking, was the same across the whole school sector (not only in schools for the deaf).
2. There are five special schools for deaf and hard of hearing students in Sweden that follow the Special School Curriculum (there is one additional special school for severely learning disabled deaf and hard of hearing students and for students who are born deaf-blind). There are also two nongovernmental schools with some classes with deaf children and children with cochlear implants. There are also six schools for hard of hearing children; these children also can attend congregated settings or "hearing classes" in ordinary schools or can be individually integrated in regular schools.

REFERENCES

Ahlgren, I. 1984. Döva barn och skriven svenska [Deaf children and written Swedish]. Forskning om Teckenspråk XIII (Sign language and the learning of Swedish by deaf children). Stockholms universitet, Institutionen för ligvistik (in Swedish).

Ahlström, M., and K. Svartholm. 1998. Barndomshörselskadades erfarenheter och upplevelser av tvåspråkighet. En pilotstudie [Experiences of bilingualism among adults, hard of hearing from childhood. A pilot study], Forskning om Teckenspråk XXI, Stockholms universitet, Institutionen för lingvistik (in Swedish).

Bellugi, U. 1980. Clues from the similarities between signed and spoken language. In *Signed and spoken language: Biological constraints on linguistic forms: Dahlem Konferenzen 1980*, ed. U. Bellugi and M. Studdert-Kennedy, 115–40. Wienhem: Verlag Chemie GmbH.

Bergman, B. 1979. Dövas teckenspråk: En inledning [Sign Language of the Deaf: An introduction], Forskning om Teckenspråk III, Stockholms universitet, Institutionen för lingvistik (in Swedish).

———. 1982. Några satstyper i det svenska teckenspråket [Some sentence types in Swedish Sign Language], Forskning om Teckenspråk XI, Stockholms universitet, Institutionen för lingvistik (in Swedish).

———. 1990. Grammaticalization of location. In *SLR '87: Papers from the Fourth International Symposium on Sign Language Research, Lappeenranta, Finland, July 15–19, 1987*, ed. W. M. Edmondson and F. Karlsson, 37–56. Hamburg: Signum-Verlag.

Cummins, J. 1996. *Negotiating identities: Education for empowerment in a diverse society.* Ontario: California Association for Bilingual Education.

Engberg-Pedersen, E. 1993. *Space in Danish Sign Language: The semantics and morphosyntax of the use of space in a visual language.* Vol. 19 of *International studies on sign language and communication of the deaf.* Hamburg: Signum-Verlag.

Fishman, J. 1965. Who speaks what language to whom and when? *La Linguistique* 2: 67–88.

———. 1972. Domains between micro- and macrosociolinguistics. In *Directions in sociolinguistics: The ethnography of communication*, ed. J. Gumperz and D. Hymes, 435–53. New York: Holt, Rinehart and Winston.

FUNKIS. 1998. FUNKIS: Funktionshindrade elever i skolan [FUNKIS: Disabled students in school], Statens Offentliga Utredningar 1998:66, Utbildnings-departementet [Swedish Ministry of Education and Science], Stockholm.

Henning, L. 2003. Syllabuses in a bilingual setting. Paper presented at EDDE: European Days of Deaf Education, May 8–11, Örebro, Sweden.

Hjulstad, O., A.-E. Kristoffersen, and E. Simonsen. 2002. *Kommunikative praksiser i barnehagen* [Communicative praxises in the preschool]. Skådalen Publication Series 17. Oslo, Norway: Skådalen Resource Centre, Norwegian Support System for Special Education (in Norwegian).

LGr 80. 1980. *Läroplan för grundskolan. Allmän del* [Curriculum for the compulsory school. General part]. Stockholm: Skolöverstyrelsen, Liber UtbildningsFörlaget.

LGr 80 Spec. 1983. *Supplement till LGr 80, Läroplan för specialskolan. Kompletterande föreskrifter till LGr 80* [Supplement to LGr 80, Curriculum for the Special School, Additional directions]. Stockholm: Skolöverstyrelsen, Liber Utbildnings-Förlaget.

Liddell, S. 2003. *Grammar, gesture and meaning in American Sign Language.* Cambridge: Cambridge University Press.

LPO 94. 1994. *Läroplan för det obligatoriska skolväsendet, förskoleklassen och fritids-hemmet 1994 (Curriculum for the compulsory school, the preschool class and the after school centre).* Stockholm: Utbildningsdepartementet.

Mahshie, S. N. 1995. *Educating deaf children bilingually: With insights and applications from Sweden and Denmark.* Washington, D.C.: Gallaudet University Press.

Proposition 1998/99:105. Elever med funktionshinder—ansvar för utbildning och stöd [Students with disabilities—responsibility for education and support]. Regeringens proposition, 6 maj 1999, Stockholm [The Swedish Parliament].

Skolverket. 1996. Specialskolan: Kursplaner, timplaner, betygskriterier och kommentarer. [The Special School: Syllabuses, timetables, grading criteria and comments]. Stockholm: The Swedish National Agency for Education.

———. 2001. Specialskola Syllabuses. http://www3.skolverket.se/ki/eng/spec_eng.pdf.

Specialskolemyndigheten [SPM; National Agency for Special Schools for the Deaf and Hard of Hearing]. 2004. Delåsrapport [Financial report]. Örebro, Sweden: Author.

———. 2004a. Kvalitetsredovisning 2004. [Quality account 2004]. Örebro, Sweden: Author.

———. 2004b. Schools for Deaf and Hard of Hearing in Sweden. http://www.spm.se/inenglish.4.b32ed4f916633f9b7fff1265.html

Kvalitetsredovisning 2004. [Quality account 2004]. Örebro, Sweden: Author.

Svartholm, K. 1993. Bilingual education for the deaf in Sweden. *Sign Language Studies* 81: 291–332.

Svartholm, K., R. Andersson, and U. Lindahl. 1993. Samspråk i dövundervisning: Studier av klassrumskommunikation i två olika skolformer för döva [Conversation in deaf education: Studies of classroom communication within two different types of schools for the deaf], Stockholms universitet, Institutionen för nordiska språk (in Swedish).

Swedish National Association for the Deaf (SDR). 1996. Handlingsprogram [Action program]. Leksand, Sweden: Sveriges Dövas Riksförbund.

United Nations (UN). 1993. *Standard rules on the equalization of opportunities for persons with disabilities*, Resolution 48/96, General Assembly, December 20, 1993. http://www.un.org/esa/socdev/enable/dissre00.htm

8

A STUDY OF NORWEGIAN DEAF AND HARD OF HEARING CHILDREN: EQUALITY IN COMMUNICATION INSIDE AND OUTSIDE FAMILY LIFE

Hilde Haualand and Inger Lise Skog Hansen

In the past, the only option for Norwegian parents was to send their deaf or hard of hearing child to a school for deaf students, and the school made the decision with respect to the language (or languages) of instruction. Hearing aids were an option only for children with some residual hearing, and parents were rarely offered the opportunity to learn sign language. With the introduction of cochlear implantation, the need to make tough choices on behalf of one's child is further heightened. In addition, parents face still more stress and uncertainty as they encounter a field in which specialists do not speak with consensus about whether implants are necessary or how children who have been implanted should be followed up on after surgery. This chapter draws on interviews with deaf and hard of hearing youth and their parents who belong to the first generation of deaf children in Norway whose parents learned sign language on an extensive basis.

When Deaf or hard of hearing children are born, their parents are now faced with numerous options. The alternatives available to them with respect to technology, language, and the education of their children have grown steadily. Knowledge of and insight into the structure and benefits of sign languages have increased considerably. That knowledge parallels the explosion in development of technical hearing devices such as hearing aids and cochlear implants. Added to this knowledge and technology is the increased emphasis on the "normalization" of the lives of disabled people and those of Deaf and hard of hearing people through integration and inclusion in the institutions and organizations of the wider society.

Could those who struggle with the agony of choices today benefit from the experiences of a generation of Deaf and hard of hearing children who are now on the threshold of adulthood? The parents of the Deaf and hard of hearing youth who were interviewed in the research project "Children of the Normalizing Ideology," (Haualand, Grønningsæter, and Skog Hansen 2003) reported in this chapter, faced a range of choices with respect to language, family communication, and school placement that is similar to what parents face today. The key difference was that, for parents of those in the research project, cochlear implantation was not as widespread when their children were born in the mid-1980s. One of the youths we interviewed, however, did receive a cochlear implant in childhood. Because of an accident, the implant was removed when she was eleven years old. Some of the youth interviewed in the project are profoundly Deaf, some function in several situations as a hard of hearing person, whereas others have only mild hearing loss. Their views of family life and, in particular, communication at home vary greatly and reflect a variety of decisions made and strategies used for including the child in the family or for coping with a child's hearing loss.

In this chapter, we focus on family involvement, communication, and relationships through the eyes of these young people. They belong to the first generation of deaf children in Norway whose parents have been encouraged to learn sign language on an extensive basis. The national program for teaching sign language to parents of deaf children was fully launched after the informants in this project were in their early teens. Their parents, nevertheless, had been offered courses in sign language and would have been strongly encouraged to learn sign language in classes offered by the local Deaf club or at the school for the Deaf their child would later attend. The young people's experiences of family life, therefore, may be quite different from the experiences of family relationships of earlier generations of Deaf people. We show how inclusion and communication strategies in the families appears to have had significant consequences for the way these youth position themselves in the world on entering adulthood.

THE PROJECT: METHODS AND RESULTS

The project "Children of the Normalizing Ideology" (Haualand, Grønningsæter, and Skog Hansen 2003) provides an initial look at particular aspects of the living conditions of Norwegian Deaf and hard of hearing people ages sixteen to twenty years. The study and the methods were exploratory because there was little previous knowledge or data on this group's living conditions and quality of life. A questionnaire was sent to all Deaf and hard of hearing students in secondary schools for Deaf students or in schools with special programs or classes for hearing impaired students in Norway. From a total of 152 possible respondents, we received seventy-seven questionnaires, a response rate of 52 percent. The surveys were sent to all schools and therefore gave us potential access to the whole population of Deaf and hard of hearing students in Norway; however, the actual response rate was low enough that the results should not be considered a representative sample. Examples from the quantitative survey that we consider instructive, however, are used to discuss the situation of Deaf and hard of hearing people in Norway (for more information and results, see Haualand, Grønningsæter, and Hansen 2003). The main data collected in the study were qualitative interviews with thirteen Deaf and hard of hearing informants. As a part of the project design, we met and conducted two semistructured interviews with each young person. These youth were at the threshold of adult life, and an explicit goal of this study was to see how they and their lives evolved in the two years between interviews. The first interviews were conducted from March to May 2002, and the second interviews from January to May 2004. The focus of our discussion here is the youths' identification and language use. The longitudinal aspect of this study offers unique access to information about the development and growth of a group of young Deaf and hard of hearing youth.

The answers with respect to identity and language in the survey guided the compilation of questions for the semistructured interviews and provided a direction for data analysis. One key question about identity posed in the questionnaire was "What would you most often label yourself?" Thirty respondents (39 percent) defined themselves as "Deaf," and forty-six (60 percent) defined themselves as "hard of hearing or hearing impaired." When asked about the medical reason for their hearing loss, 37 percent said they did not know. Given that such a large group was uncertain about the extent of their hearing loss, we decided to investigate the idea of self-identification rather than reported hearing loss. The lack of knowledge about the extent of their loss also provided us with a strong indication that the identity label was more important to the young people surveyed than the extent of their hearing loss.

In analyzing and reporting the data, we take a social constructivist perspective on identities and identification. The youth themselves, not their ears, are the foremost crafters of their own identities. Almost all the youth supported the discourse prevalent in the Deaf rights movement that deaf people belong to a linguistic and cultural minority, not a disability group (agreed to by almost 90 percent of those labeling themselves Deaf), and 80 percent of those labeling themselves hard of hearing agree that Deaf people's language competence seems to be intimately connected with self-identification. A total of 91 percent of those identifying themselves as hard of hearing or hearing impaired said Norwegian was their best language whereas 80 percent of those describing themselves as Deaf considered Norwegian Sign Language (Norsk tegnspråk) to be their best language. Approximately 80 percent of all respondents know both Norwegian Sign Language and Norwegian (written, spoken, or both) and are therefore at least bilingual. The question of "preferred language" did not pertain to which language they had learned first or used the most, but to which language they considered their preferred language or the language in which they themselves felt they functioned best.

At the time of the interviews, most of the respondents lived at home (60 percent) and saw one or both parents every day. Twenty percent lived in dormitories at school, and the rest lived alone or with friends or partners. A little more than 60 percent have no other Deaf or hard of hearing family members, 19 percent have Deaf or hard of hearing siblings, and about 10 percent have Deaf or hard of hearing parents. The last statistic is consistent with the "rule of thumb" widely held in the deafness field that approximately 90 percent of all hearing impaired children are born into hearing families who, in all likelihood, know no sign language and generally lack insight into the consequences of congenital hearing loss. Less than half the youth (42 percent) reported having hearing family members who used signed language at home. This percentage is not surprising. The parents of the youth in this study who undertook sign language training did so in their leisure time, usually from the school for the deaf their child later attended or from the local Deaf club. Although parents in Norway, for almost two decades, have been encouraged to learn sign language, a formal program for teaching and supporting parents' acquisition of sign language began only in 1996. Since the introduction of this program, the parents of youth in this study have been eligible for two weeks sign language instruction per year. Table 8.1 shows that of those who stated that Norwegian Sign Language is their best language, 76 percent said that sign language was the language used at home (this percentage includes the respondents who have Deaf parents).

Table 8.1. Language used at home and "best" personal language

Language Used at Home	Best Language: Norwegian/ Spoken Language		Best Language: NTS/ Sign Language		Total	
	n	%	n	%	n	%
Norwegian	34	79	9	21	43	100
Norwegian Sign Language (NTS)	5	24	16	76	21	100
All	39	61	25	39	64	100

These numbers indicate that the language barrier that has traditionally existed between Deaf young people and their hearing families has weakened and that more Deaf and hard of hearing children are growing up with sign language in the home than previous generations. In the past, the only children who grew up using sign language in the home were those children with Deaf parents and the few whose hearing parents had sufficient resources to learn Norwegian Sign Language by their own initiative. However, policy has shifted from one that supported unilaterally trying to teach deaf and hard of hearing children to speak their parents' language to one that supported teaching the parents their child's (potential) language. As the insight into and understanding of the significance of sign language has increased in Norway, the social pressure for parents to learn sign language if their child is deaf or hard of hearing has intensified significantly. This pressure started before Norway launched one of the world's most comprehensive education programs for parents of children who use sign language in 1996. All parents of deaf or hard of hearing children born after 1992 are entitled to receive at least forty weeks free instruction in Norwegian Sign Language and Deaf culture before the child reaches the age of sixteen (Liltved 2002). In addition, the parents of children born earlier than 1992 are offered two weeks instruction in Norwegian Sign Language annually until their child reaches sixteen. The youth interviewed in this project were all born before 1992, and therefore, their parents were provided with the second option. Still, 42 percent of the youth reported that sign language was used at home, which is an indication that many parents made the effort to learn sign language before the formal establishment of a parent program.

Key differences are apparent between those youth who experienced relatively seamless communication between home and school and those who struggled to be included in the family because their parents had not learned signed language. Generally, but not exclusively, those who felt included in the family had parents who had learned to sign. Others who had parents who did not sign at all could still feel included, but they asked more questions about identity and belonging than those who had families where signs were used.

Quite "Ordinary" Youth

The current generation of Deaf people has quite a different experience of growing up deaf or hard of hearing than the generations before them. They have experienced an increase in the general acceptance of deafness and an accompanying reduction in the stigma attached to it, the wider knowledge about the legitimacy of native sign languages, and the change in education programs. The increased visibility of sign language in public life, especially on television and through the use of interpreters, has reduced the traditional stigma attached to Deaf people and their native sign languages. Through sign language interpreters, accessibility for to Deaf people is secured in more arenas than ever before. Telephones with text messages, Internet chat rooms, and e-mail are also regularly used among Deaf youth, which reduces the communication barriers.

When asked to present their view of themselves at the beginning of the interviews, many of the youth emphasized concepts such as normality, being like everyone else, and being ordinary:

> My name is Oline, I am born deaf. I am unemployed, and have dreams, like everyone else. (Oline, age twenty-one, interview two)

> * * *

> I am Mia, a Deaf girl. Newlywed, kind, nice, bad, want to quit smoking, have positive and negative sides, just like everyone else. (Mia, age twenty-two, interview two)

> * * *

> If I shall present myself for the other students in my class or for someone here in school, I mean, for hearing people, I would say that I am an ordinary girl. (Helene, age eighteen, interview two)

> * * *

> I am Jon, an ordinary boy from Kristiansand. (Jon, age twenty, interview two)

> * * *

> My name is Marianne, and I am eighteen years old. My interests are clothes, art and other ordinary interests, like most other youth have. (Marianne, age eighteen, interview two)

Some participants did not know what to say; they said they felt so ordinary that there was really not much to tell. But at the same time, many such as Oline, Mia, and Helene, above, included reference to a Deaf identity or some other aspect of hearing loss. In another example, Tone said:

> My name is Tone, I am twenty years old and I come from a small town in western Norway. I am a student and I have had a hearing aid since I was ten years old. (Tone, age twenty, interview two)

This insistence on being "ordinary" or "just like everyone else" could testify to some awareness that other people may perceive them as different or special.

But there is also some resistance to the distinction between "special" and "normal," as Marianne explains:

> Deaf people are a cultural minority, but also a part of something larger. It is a bit provocative when people who claim they are "normal" say that we are special, when we really are like them. (Marianne, age sixteen, interview one)

Marianne captures very well the response of many of the Deaf and hard of hearing young participants in the project. She perceives herself as an ordinary girl who lives a life just like any other person her age. In her eyes, she is quite ordinary, but with individual dreams and personal plans. The youth interviewed in this study discussed their deafness or hearing loss as just one of many facets of their personality. Despite this view, most (perhaps with the exception of those born into Deaf families) identified as feeling more or less "different" since their hearing loss was diagnosed. The key question is not whether, in our eyes, their difference is "special" or "normal," but how the youth and their families handled and continue to negotiate this difference.

INCLUSION, INTEGRATION, OR EXCLUSION?

Some of the youth in this study grew up in families that did not use sign language. Consequently, they had only recently started to interact with other Deaf and hard of hearing people. Others of the youth had grown up in a sign language environment and were facing the challenges of negotiating as an adult in a nonsigning world. The transitions experienced by the youth are discussed in this section.

First and foremost, the youth reveal in their accounts that identity as being Deaf or hard of hearing is not a fixed attribute; it is a way of becoming rather than a way of being. They were on the threshold of adult life and were going through, or facing, great changes in their lives. They were leaving the protected life within their families and establishing a life of their own in social environments that may be quite different from home. Their childhood experiences and what they had learned about being Deaf or hard of hearing would influence how they interact with people outside the homes in which they had grown up. This personal background would influence the way they would craft their lives as young Deaf or hard of hearing adults.

Experiences of Inclusion

Hanne and Maja are two of the girls who grew up in a family with hearing parents and siblings who learned sign language to communicate with them, and they were educated through sign language. Therefore, they have grown up surrounded by sign language at school and at home, contexts where they have experienced equality in terms of communication. Their challenge now is to find ways to communicate and interact extensively with those who are not familiar with Deaf people or sign language.

In the first interview with Hanne (age seventeen), she said that the signing milieu at home gave her a sense of equality and belonging:

> I know I am very lucky to have such a supportive family as mine. They have all learned sign language, and I have never got any special treatment at home because I am Deaf. (Hanne, age seventeen, interview one)

When Hanne was young, her parents, siblings and grandparents went to a county college for the Deaf for six months to learn Norwegian Sign Language. The story Hanne tells about herself is one of inclusion and participation through sign language. She attended a school for Deaf students throughout elementary and secondary school and attended a class with all hearing co-students for the first time when she entered college. When she had been ready to start secondary school, she had considered attending a school with all hearing pupils but had decided on a school for Deaf students, even if it meant that courses of primary interest to her could not be offered:

> I like art, but the upper secondary school for the Deaf does not offer that subject. There would be more choices at a public upper secondary school and a larger social milieu. But I'd rather not be the only Deaf pupil at a large hearing school. I feel that the Deaf school gives me more (Hanne, age seventeen, interview one)

Her choice of higher education was motivated by her ambition to make a career in the arts. For the first time in her life, she had to interact with nonsigning hearing people on an everyday basis.

> It was a big change to enter a school with only hearing people. In the beginning, I felt I did not have the freedom to say what I wanted to. And I could not participate how I wanted. I was only able to communicate through the interpreter, and it was hard to say anything. Several times, they had finished talking before I entered the discussion. And someone else had already said what I said. But I just had to be patient. Things gradually improved. The other students also learned to calm down, show consideration, talk one at a time and so on. We also decided that they should learn one new sign every day, but now we communicate fine, so we don't do that anymore. (Hanne, age nineteen, interview two)

At the time of the second interview, Hanne told me she was mostly with hearing people who knew sign language. Most of her Deaf friends from school had moved to other cities to work or study. She said, however, that she had always been around both Deaf and hearing people, so this situation was really nothing new to her. At the same time, she recognized that she was not becoming completely immersed in a hearing world:

> I am more relaxed with Deaf people. I can be myself and say exactly what I want. With hearing people, everything becomes a bit more circumstantial.

I use more time to say what I want and also often leave out quite a lot. (Hanne, age nineteen, interview two)

Hanne appeared confident and gave the impression that she had considerable social resources. She had never been isolated or excluded from social interaction with her family or peers. She was aware of the huge change in her life when she entered college—being the only deaf person in her classes and having to interact with hearing people who did not know sign language on an everyday and extensive basis. When discussing which upper secondary school she had decided she should attend, she expressed that she had been aware of the challenges communicating with those who do not use signed language. Nevertheless, growing up in a signing environment did not necessarily make her less prepared for interaction with those who do not sign. Rather, it appears that her experience of being "part of a group" has given her the social skills needed to join any other group. She has learned how to modify her behavior and make other people modify their own so she can participate in a full social life with hearing people who do not know Norwegian Sign Language. Hanne has well-established relationships with hearing people: with her hearing family and a hearing boyfriend whom she has taught sign language. Being born into a hearing family, she has been intimately exposed to a hearing world from birth. She reflected on this experience in the first interview:

I reckon that I will be part of both the hearing and Deaf world. I need both milieus and there are no big differences between hearing people and Deaf people. (Hanne, age seventeen, interview one)

Maja is also the only Deaf child in a family of hearing signers. She stated, "Deaf and hearing are really the same; they are alike" (Maja, age sixteen, interview one). Hanne and Maja's statements are illustrative of the new generation of multicultural young Deaf people in Norway. They are confident in their identity as Deaf people, and they relate well to hearing people. Their self-confidence and belief that they may be different but "just as good" seems to give them the assertiveness needed to demand the right to full participation in a hearing society. During the first interviews, they could not remember any incidences at home marking them as "special" or deviant in their home setting. Both said they felt just like any other family member, a view that reflects their subjective position that, in general, they can relate to both Deaf and hearing people. The "normal" family bonds seem to have influenced the development of their worldview. Neither girl has been put under pressure to "integrate" into a structure in which she did not fit. Rather, their closest surroundings transformed to fit their needs. As a consequence, they did not question their belonging, position, identity, or rights.

The Integration Experience

Helene, age sixteen at the first interview and eighteen at the second interview, alternates between describing herself as Deaf and as hard of hearing and confesses that her self-image is changing. She grew up in a hearing family, and only her mother used some signs. Helene describes herself as being the "different" child, the child who is not like her siblings.

> I am quite left out, compared to my sisters. I am in one sense one of them, but there have always been problems with me who am hard of hearing. I do not understand what they are talking about when we are eating dinner. I appreciate my mom using voice and signs, and that she shows me some consideration. Still, I feel left out, and I am quarrelling a lot with my little sister since there are so many misunderstandings. I have always been the bad girl at home, while my big sister is so calm and I look up to her. I have always felt left out at home. (Helene, age sixteen, interview one)

Her description of social relationships and her feelings when communicating with other people outside her home resemble the communication situation in her family. She did not quite fit in anywhere, feeling left out with both hearing and Deaf people.

> I do not feel that I fit in neither with Deaf or hearing people. Deaf people use sign language so much and so fast, that I often feel more hearing than Deaf. But, I do not understand what hearing people are saying, and I was often tired and in a bad mood when I had been with hearing people. One and one is okay, but not many at a time. My mother wanted me to participate more in the Deaf club, but I did not quite like it there. (Helene, age sixteen, interview one)

In the same interview, she added:

> I feel that I am becoming more and more Deaf but, to be honest, I must admit that I miss hearing people. I belong to both worlds, but I also fall between two worlds. I am concerned with finding my place, to learn who I am. (Helene, age sixteen, interview one)

Two years later, in the second interview, Helene again told us about identity in progress—but now also identity in retrospect:

> When I am with Deaf people, I feel like I am Deaf. It can be a problem to be hard of hearing. One falls between two worlds, one does not always know where one belongs. This was much more of a problem to me before, especially when I was about fourteen years old. At that time, I was continuously in search of myself and who I was. That was one of my reasons for going to Bergen and a secondary school for the Deaf there. I wanted to find out more about myself. Now, I don't feel the same need for searching anymore. I can choose both milieus, and in that manner it is an advantage to be hard of hearing. But I feel more comfortable when I am with Deaf people. I can relax and don't need any remedies to understand what is going on. With hearing people, I need technical aids and it is more constraints and lots of "what did you say?" (Helene, age eighteen, interview two)

Helene lived in Bergen for only a year before she moved home again for a variety of reasons. One reason seemed to be that her parents were not quite satisfied with her school work and wanted her to live at home so they could follow her more closely. In both interviews, she emphasized her closeness to her father and how her parents encourage her to strive for an excellent education and a good career. At the second interview, she was attending a large upper secondary school with only a few other hard of hearing students, none of whom were in her class.

The year in Bergen, when she was almost exclusively with Deaf people, seems to have been some help in her search for herself. Having grown up in a hearing family with little signing and only sporadic contact with other Deaf sign language users, the year in Bergen was her first intensive meeting with sign language users. When she left Bergen, for the first time she was able to compare two different language environments—signing and nonsigning—and position herself in relation to these. In Bergen, she found people who in one way or another shared her "visual horizon." They communicated in a way that demanded less attention from her, and eventually, she found "free space" where she could relax and communicate at the same time. It appears that this change in social environment caused some changes in her way of viewing herself. Helene's experience is an example of the close interaction between social milieu and processes of personal identity. Helene knows her position in both worlds and has decided that she is able, and wants, to take advantage of each. She makes frequent visits to Bergen to see Deaf friends and sometimes meets with other Deaf young people in her hometown. But she also maintains some close friendships with hearing people with whom she socializes on an everyday basis and goes out partying.

To many, crafting a sound identity as a young adult and a Deaf or hard of hearing person is an ambiguous task. Questions of belonging to the Deaf or hearing worlds seem to add pressure to the anxiety often connected to the teenage years. Helene seems to have handled the transition between Deaf and hearing surroundings well and has found a place within both worlds. Yet other young people interviewed in this study seemed to struggle more with these issues of belonging and family relationships.

Exclusion within the Family

Frode and Oline are two of the youth who have grown up in a situation typical of a time when the hearing parents of deaf and hard of hearing children were not given the opportunity to learn sign language. Neither of their parents learned any signs beyond some simple, natural gestures. Both Oline and Frode can use their voices and hearing aids to communicate in spoken Norwegian in some situations, but neither find that this approach is sufficient for full social interaction with other people. Both have negative experiences from home of situations and a climate that did not recognize their needs as hard of hearing members of their families. Frode's story is an example of a deaf person who feels left out in his own family. He comments in his first interview:

> I am not very close to my siblings. They were all talking at once. Even though
> I asked them again and again what they were talking about. I often ran away

and walked out for hours. Or I sat in my room listening to music. (Frode, age twenty, interview one)

Two years later, at the time of the second interview, he had finished vocational school, had moved back to his hometown, and was employed in a sheltered workshop. Some of his work colleagues knew some signs, but he was totally left out at meetings at work because of a shortage of interpreters where he lives. He said he had little contact with his family, explaining,

Nobody in my family knows sign language. They say it is not necessary, but that is not true. They don't want to learn it. My brother used to be a little interested, but he was so much out fishing, and now it is too late. They know simple signs for eating, go out, and so forth. It is just as hard to communicate with them, as it was earlier. They do not respect me and they ignore me. They tell me it is up to me to speak up, but that is not easy when I feel bad. (Frode, age twenty-two, interview two)

Frode has a hearing girlfriend whom he met through an Internet chat room. They plan to rent an apartment together, and he is teaching her some signs. During his years at the vocational school for the Deaf, he was ostracized by some of the other students and became friends with very few people. Norwegian is still his first language, but he learned quite a lot of sign language at the vocational school. He says:

Norwegian is my best language. And sign language! I miss other Deaf people, to relax [with]. With my girlfriend, I use sign language a bit, since I do not want to forget it. (Frode, age twenty-two, interview two)

Frode seems to feels that he does not belong anywhere. The other Deaf pupils at the vocational school did not accept him, he is not able to follow meetings and discussions at work, and he does not feel accepted within his own family. Other than when he is with his girlfriend, it seems as though he has no "free space" where he can fully participate on his own terms. Neither his production nor understanding of sign language is good enough to interact, without constraints, with other sign language users. His chance of following a sound-based conversation with other people is unlikely. It is not possible to predict his future, but his way toward adulthood and developing an image of totality seems far thornier and ambiguous than for Helene and several of the other youth interviewed in the study. When asked his thoughts about his hearing loss, he gave a negative message:

I do not like to be hard of hearing. It is better to be hearing. I do not understand what people are talking about. If the physicians find a cure, I want to become hearing. I do not feel well with Deaf people, it is better to be with hearing people. (Frode, age twenty, interview one)

His view of his own hearing loss seems to reflect the negative feedback he has received from his home, school, and work environments. He feels that his parents have never fully recognized his needs, nor have other signed language users accepted him for who he is.

Oline's parents also never learned signed language. Unlike Frode, however, she went to schools where the teachers used either signed Norwegian or Norwegian Sign Language, and she has a sound footing within the community of signed language users. At the first interview, she described the tough conditions in her family:

> I often experienced that I was left out at home, not many people there knew any sign language. My parents failed to take care of me, and the probation officers thought that there was a lot of abuse at home. I did things that were not quite common. For example, I smashed a lot of items and was often angry. I believe I did that to get attention. It was so lonely to be the only deaf person in the family, but when I started to smash things and behave badly, they at least saw me, and I got a scolding. I started to smoke to make them see me. (Oline, age twenty, interview one)

For some time, Oline had very little contact with her family. The relationship with her parents seemed quite constrained at the time of the first interview. By the second interview, two years later, Oline said that much had changed over the past year, including the way she viewed her communication capabilities and use of sign language. She had decided to stop using hearing aids and to use sign language much more extensively than earlier. This decision brought on further conflict with her family:

> Sign language is more important to me, but my family thought it was silly that I did not want to use speech. We had many conflicts for a while, and we had no contact. I told them they would lose me if they did not respect me. But after an incident at home, my father realised how little my hearing aid actually helped me and how little use I really had of my voice, when I really cannot control how loud I speak. After a while, he sent me an e-mail where he wrote that he respected my choice, understood why I had made my decision and also said he understood why I almost never participated in family parties and so on. That e-mail really meant a lot to me. They will always be my family, so I was glad to receive that e-mail. (Oline, age twenty-two, interview two)

Oline's sound footing in an environment of sign language users and her relationship with her Deaf boyfriend gave her a position from which she could speak out against her family and make some (communicative) demands on them. Oline did not find inclusion in her family environment but eventually achieved it among her friends.

Helene and Frode grew up in a hearing, Norwegian-speaking environment, learning about the Deaf community in their late teens. Oline always had the Deaf community there. Their reflections and experiences from their upbringings are very different, but all of them give the message that they have had to (or still) struggle to find places where they can belong. Their parents may have assumed that their children could hear so well that sign language was not necessary for family communication, or they may not have had the opportunity or resources to learn Norwegian Sign Language. Oral communication on a one-to-one basis may have functioned fairly well, but it had not allowed them to take part in the spontaneous and intimate communication often taken for granted in a family setting.

Helene and Oline also give an impression of being confident young women. Even though Helene feels that her family have been careful to include her most of the time, she talks about the feeling of being a special member in her own family. Oline had a network of Deaf friends and, later, teachers who showed her a way of communicating that works best for her; she had the confidence and personal resources to tell her family what she needed. Frode, in contrast, experienced significant exclusion from his family, which makes him reluctant to have much contact with them now. At the same time, he was not given the opportunity to learn sign language well and, therefore, also experiences exclusion from the one place he potentially could fit in. Unlike other informants who grew up with parents using sign language, the question of belonging or self-identity did not arise for Oline, Helene, and Frode as a "matter of course." For Oline, Helene, and Frode, the experience of being a "special" member in their own families seemed to add ambiguity and anxiety to the process of developing an identity as a teenager or young adult.

Acceptance for Being Themselves

The youths' views about hearing loss, identity, and family relationships seem to reflect not only their experiences of being treated as either equal or unequal members of their families but also the extent of their struggle to communicate with those who should be closest to them. Unlike earlier generations, over the past decade, many Norwegian parents who have deaf and hard of hearing children have learned Norwegian Sign Language and use it for family communication. Generally, the Deaf or hard of hearing children in these families are included in family life and communication from an early age. As young adults, these youth reject an inferior or deficit status within their family and expect or demand to be treated on equal terms outside the family. Parents' acceptance of their child's deafness, represented by their own acquisition of sign language, contributed to a high level of confidence in these youth to see themselves as Deaf people.

Much of the earlier focus within deaf education has been on teaching Deaf and hard of hearing children to speak. The mindset was that this approach enabled them to communicate with their families and the surrounding (hearing) world. As Ladd (2003) writes, they were perceived as potential hearing children who could not hear. With the perspective of Freire (1970, 55), it is clear that there has been an attempt to position these children within a structure that made them "beings for others." For some, communication on a one-to-one basis may have functioned well, but it did not allow them to take part in the spontaneous and intimate communication often taken for granted in a family setting. Teaching Norwegian Sign Language to parents of Deaf and hard of hearing children seems to have helped families overcome barriers. The youth consider themselves as insiders and expect to be treated as such, even within a hearing society.

The results of this study challenge the view that cochlear implantation and a unilateral focus on speech development for deaf or hard of hearing children is necessary for full family communication. Indeed, we found that the parents who learned sign language, and who used it at home when their child was present, changed the structure of the family environment to fit the needs of their child. This approach allowed their children to become "beings for themselves" (Freire 1970, 55) and to function on their own terms. It stands to reason to expect that those who have experienced full access to family life will not accept limited access to society in their adult life. Many have experienced being insiders in their families, and they expect to be treated as insiders in a hearing society, too. Several of the Deaf and hard of hearing young people interviewed in this study perceive themselves as participants in a variety of social situations and contexts, in both the hearing and Deaf worlds. In practice, many of them are reuniting two worlds that, traditionally, have been divided by language barriers.

REFERENCES

Freire, P. 1970. *Pedagogy of the oppressed*. New York: Penguin Books.

Haualand, H., A. Grønningsæter, and I. L. Skog Hansen. 2003. Uniting divided worlds—A study of deaf and hard of hearing youth, Fafo report 412, Fafo, Oslo, Norway. http://www.fafo.no/pub/rapp/412/412.pdf.

Ladd, P. 2003. *Understanding deaf culture: In search of deafhood*. Clevedon, United Kingdom: Multilingual Matters.

Liltved, B. S. 2002. Tegnspråkopplæring for foreldre til døve og sterkt tunghørte barn, Statens Utdanningskontor i Aust-Agder [Sign language training for parents of deaf and hard of hearing children]. Aust-Agder, Norway: State Educational Agency.

9

FREEDOM OF SPEECH FOR DEAF PEOPLE

Paal Richard Peterson

This chapter discusses some of the educational and human rights issues that arise if focus is placed solely on the oral education of children with cochlear implants without giving priority to those children's access to information. The author questions how deaf people's freedom of speech can be secured and whether they can be said to be active participants in a democratic society if cochlear implantation does not give deaf people perfect hearing and disallows the use of native sign language.

COCHLEAR IMPLANTATION IS HERE TO STAY

In Scandinavian countries, as in other countries around the world, we have experienced a great increase in the number of cochlear implantation operations for deaf children. In Norway, about 90 percent of children who are born deaf and a growing number of deaf adults are now receiving cochlear implants. In my view, we need to accept that cochlear implants and other technologies are here to stay. Rather than debate the pros and cons of implantation, we need to discuss the more relevant issue concerning which educational approach will best support an implanted child's development: a purely oral education, simultaneous use of speech and a contrived signed system, or native sign language? Methodological disagreements among teachers of deaf children have taken place for more than a century; with the introduction of cochlear implants, we are witnessing yet another controversy over deaf education. In a discussion in the Norwegian parliament in 1899, Christian Knudsen, a member of the parliament, stated:

> The situation is that among teachers of the deaf we see a great deal of disagreement. Here in the parliament we can hear that our committee [the Church Committee] often disagrees about different cases. The honoured members of this parliament should really know how much teachers of the deaf and the people who know much about deaf education disagree. They would find that in comparison the Church Committee is a really peaceful place. (cited in Bjørndal 1981, 26)

The situation has not changed very much since then. We are now experiencing a greater degree of polarization between oralists and signers than has been seen in the past ten to twenty years. For the past two decades, Norwegian Sign

Language has been recognized as fundamental to the education of deaf and hard of hearing children in Norway and included in the national curriculum. With the latest cochlear implant technologies, we face a situation in which some people have so strong a belief in cochlear implants that they want to remove sign language from educational programs for deaf children with cochlear implants.

The controversy over educational methods—oralism or sign language—is often characterized as a pendulum, swinging first in one direction and then the other. I regard this characterization as a pessimistic view that leaves almost nothing to the actions of individuals or to the collective knowledge of society. To move forward, we need a new perspective. Instead of eternally shifting direction, we must say: "We now have knowledge that they did not have 100 or 150 years ago." The controversy then becomes more like a spiral with a narrowing top, the two paradigms moving ever closer together.

If the situation is that all implant recipients can hear quite well, then why should they have the need for sign language? Even if *all* deaf children are implanted, sign language is needed to ensure deaf people's freedom of speech, so they have every opportunity to give and receive information.

Article 19 of the United Nation's *Universal Declaration of Human Rights* (UN 1948) states:

> Everyone has the right to freedom of opinion and expression; this right includes freedom to hold opinions without interference and to seek, receive and impart information and ideas through any media and regardless of frontiers.

In this chapter, I focus on the significance of freedom of speech, a basic human right. It affects any situation that involves access to information, including both the right to give and to receive information. Two main purposes for providing information are to persuade and to convince. The Norwegian philosopher Hans B. Skjervheim (1968) introduced these concepts of convincing and persuading based on the ancient Greek philosophers Socrates and Plato and on the difference between *episteme* (true knowledge) and *doxa* (rhetoric). The act of persuading another person presupposes that a "subject" (the persuader) acts in relation to an "object" (the other person) that is being manipulated by the subject for his or her needs. In contrast, the act of convincing another person requires that a "subject" (S1) needs to act in relation to another "subject" (S2). Here, the goal is not to dominate another person but to convince the second subject (S2) by his or her own thoughts and feelings that the arguments used are the best ones for both S1 and S2. We can say that acting in a subject-subject relationship requires both speakers to have equal access to all the information in a given situation. If, however, one of the speakers has more knowledge and more up-to-date information than the other, then the situation is characterized as a subject-object relationship. The subject-object relationship largely describes the situation for deaf people.

Deaf People as Objects

When the society creates barriers to information access for Deaf people, for instance when there are no interpreters on television or when visual communication is avoided, then Deaf people become objects because they do not have the same access to information as their hearing counterparts.

Political Participation

A basic goal for all those involved in the education of deaf people, whether through oralism or sign language, should be to enable deaf people to be active members of society. To become active members, deaf people need knowledge, and educators need a willingness to empower them. One measure of a citizen's participation in society is to vote. Other ways of being involved in politics include using the media, participating as a member of an organization, or taking part in public protests.

Previous research of deaf people's involvement in politics in Norway (see Peterson 2001) shows that deaf individuals participate in elections less frequently than other members of Norwegian society. When 78.3 percent of the population voted in the general election in 1997, only 69 percent of the deaf people who were surveyed confirmed that they voted that year. (The actual voting percentage among deaf people is, in fact, unlikely to have exceeded 55 percent. First, we must expect an error margin up to 4 percent. Second, when people are asked questions about their behavior, they often want to place themselves in a favorable light, thereby stating that they voted even if they did not (the problem of social desirability). Third, because only 60 percent of the total sample returned the survey, it is presumable that this sample represents a selected constellation.) In my view, the most reliable explanation for the differences in voting levels among deaf and hearing people is their unequal access to information. A very small amount of all the political and economic information made available to the public is made visually accessible to deaf people through sign language interpreting or subtitling. Deaf people's limited access to information and varying levels of political literacy are two key barriers, among others, to political activism among deaf people (Bateman 1996). In addition, deaf people do not generally use the mainstream media to draw attention to their political struggles. This characterization of the Deaf community reflects the two facets of freedom of speech: receiving and producing information.

If there were no deaf people, would 100 percent of voters participate in an election? There is, of course, no direct link between access to information and voting; hearing nonvoters offer a variety of reasons for why they do not vote. Nevertheless, to make use of information, we must know how to handle it and appreciate its value. One skill that enables effective use of information is that of fully mastering a language. For deaf and hearing impaired people, sign language gives them the chance to acquire language without delay because it is not based on sound.

Another example of limited access to information is found in the voting patterns of deaf people in relation to party choice. Research has shown that deaf people are more connected to left-wing parties in Norway such as the Socialists and Social Democrats (Peterson 2001). One explanation is that the "information gap" deaf people experience makes the Labor Party a safe choice because it has traditionally been the strongest political party in Norway. Research of mainstream votes shows that about half the voting public decide who they will vote for *during* an election campaign, a practice that gives the media growing importance. Without equal access to this information, deaf people's choice of political parties becomes more unchanging because they stay with what they know.

Elections and media, however, are not the only ways to engage in politics. When we study deaf people's membership in (Deaf) organizations and participation in public protests, we find a different picture. In Norway, 76 percent of deaf people are members of a Deaf club or another Deaf organization (Peterson 2001). Deaf people also appear to take part in protests such as demonstrations and strikes more often than hearing people do. One explanation is that the protests in which the deaf people were involved were initiated by deaf people themselves and therefore have a high level of Deaf community participation. Therefore, one cannot say that Deaf people are less involved in politics than hearing people, but they do engage in politics in a different manner. Nevertheless, a key objective should be to raise the percentage of voters within the deaf community. When deaf people vote, they show that, in addition to fighting for deaf human rights through other political avenues, they also want to give their opinion on taxes, pollution, and the distribution of goods and burdens in society (Peterson 2004). This point brings us back to freedom of speech and the subject-subject form of communication. If more deaf people are to use their voting rights, then access to information needs to improve, and the society needs to avoid objectifying deaf people.

Expectations of Parents and Surroundings

Home background and, in particular, parents are the most important sources of education in a person's life. Thus, a fundamental requirement of education is good communication among family members who, generally, speak the same language. But what happens if the child is deaf and implanted and his parents expect him to hear and speak orally, as his only language?

All deaf people have experienced being the only deaf person in a hearing environment. For those in that situation, it is easy to laugh when others laugh, even if they have no idea what the joke was about (or was it a joke?). They can remain silent or follow other people as an easy escape from communication problems. I have done so myself many times. But when I act in this way, I subjugate myself because I allow hearing people to treat me as an object. I make the situation easy for them, and I avoid challenging them to improve their level of visual communication.

Many deaf people have experienced the same feeling of being an outsider and of being left out of daily conversation with hearing colleagues, students, or friends. I am afraid that children with implants will experience those same feelings if those in the surrounding environment are unaware of their situation and assume that an implanted child can comprehend all that is being said. Might these children with implants put themselves into the position of objects, appearing as if they can hear satisfactorily when in fact they cannot? Of course, the answer may be yes. All parents, regardless of how their deaf children are educated, must be aware of such situations.

When oral educators describe their educational programs, they often tell about a situation in which one child is undertaking speech and listening training with one teacher. When the child is not allowed to use any signs, at what point will this situation turn into a subject-object relationship rather than a subject-subject relationship? For how long must an implanted child accept not fully perceiving the spoken word as he undertakes training that may enable him to speak and hear later on? I have no clear answer to this question other than to be aware of how easy it is to get caught in the subject-object trap.

Deaf People as Subjects

When the society involves deaf people by making information accessible to them, then deaf people are treated like subjects and, as a consequence, they are free to act as individuals.

An Example from Football (Soccer): Improve What You Already Can Do Quite Well

One of the proudest and greatest sports stories in Norway is the success of the soccer team Rosenborg. They have been Norway's best club since 1992. During the 1990s, they participated in the European Champion League eight years in a row. The team is from Trondheim, not very far from the Polar Circle. How could a team from a city packed with snow and ice for six months of the year become a success at football? The team's manager for most of these years, Nils Arne Eggen, explains that the key to Rosenborg's success is that players improve on the skills that they have today so they can be the best tomorrow. The focus should be substantially, but not entirely, on the player's natural abilities.

This chapter is not about football, so you might wonder why I am writing about Rosenborg. I mention their philosophy because I think that key to their success can also be applied to deaf children (but not in the sense that deaf youth should be soccer players for Rosenborg—although that would be wonderful!). The key to success—for a soccer team or a deaf child—is to focus one's natural abilities. Deaf children, with or without cochlear implants, have the ability to use sight. And fortunately, there is a language based on sight. Why reject that?

If you are a hearing person reading this chapter, imagine that sound suddenly disappears. Perhaps you accompany your daughter to the railway station, show her to the train, then go and wait for the train to leave. Then you remember that you did not bring any food for her to eat during the journey, and you start shouting "Do you have anything to eat?" She cannot hear you, and in despair, you start moving your fingers to the front of your mouth and then point to your daughter. She understands, she turns to show you her backpack with food in it, and as you see her response, you calm down.

What did you just do? When the sound disappeared, you started using simple gestures, iconic signs, an easy sign language. This imaginary episode shows that when people cannot hear, they spontaneously start to use visual elements to produce and receive messages, just as deaf people do when they use sign language. It may be called a natural ability.

I do not see this focus on natural ability as excluding the development of qualities we do not already have. If that kind of exclusion were the case, then Rosenborg would have been a skiing team, not a football team. Deaf children can profit from speech and listening training, and as long as deaf people themselves want to take part in such training, it is appropriate that it continue. But if all those who have cochlear implants can hear quite well, why use sign language? I think the answer is because "quite well" is not always good enough. Cochlear implant professionals agree that an implant does not give a deaf person perfect hearing. Consequently, in some situations, cochlear implant recipients' hearing will not provide access to sufficient information to ensure they can act as fully informed citizens.

So when deaf people with cochlear implants can hear "quite well," it must be up to them what language they prefer to use when listening to one another. They may be following a televised political debate before an election and manage to hear almost everything that is said, but sometimes they miss points. If at those moments they were able to look at the sign language interpreter on the television screen, then they would comprehend all the information. They could, if provided, also read the captions (although in a debate, sign language interpreting is often superior to written captions because the interpreting takes place simultaneously with the speech).

Sign Language Programs for Parents

In Norway, parents of deaf and hearing impaired children have the option to receive sign language training. This option, a module-based program of forty weeks duration, is undertaken during the child's first sixteen years. Two main subjects are taught: Norwegian Sign Language (900 hours) and topics about parenting a deaf or hearing impaired child (100 hours). Siblings are also offered eight weeks of sign language training. The training, board, and lodging are provided free for parents, generally at government-owned resource centers. Currently, approximately 800 parents are taking part in this training (the population of Norway is about 4.5 million).

I recently surveyed these parents (723 parents were invited to participate) and found that the program is of great importance for communication within these families (Peterson 2005). As a result of the training, 88 percent of parents said they communicate better at home, 76 percent believe it provided their family with a better quality of life, and 85 percent said they never considered quitting the course. Almost all the parents who join this program, particularly those who started the training over the last few years, have children with cochlear implants. A satisfaction score based on selected questions was devised to represent parents' overall impression of the training. The satisfaction score ranged from 1 to 3, and 1 represented the best outcome. The average of all questions showed a satisfaction score of 1.46. That average gives the impression that parents are satisfied with the sign language training they are offered but that there is potential for improvement. One of the areas often mentioned is language choice because many parents want more focus on the simultaneous use of speech and sign. We have concluded that new programs must be developed to satisfy parents' needs, but without spoiling what is already available and functions well for many people (that is, native sign language).

Real Inclusion

With the issue of language choice comes the question of how to include people with different types of hearing loss in communication that takes place in a group setting or in the media. I have shown how the right to acquire information is a basic principle of freedom of speech and that lack of information may be a valid explanation for the phenomenon that deaf voters are not as active as their hearing counterparts. But what measures can be used to assess whether freedom of speech has been breached, promoting discrimination against deaf people? A solution may be to use the philosophic distinction between a subject and object, as described earlier in this chapter.

The presence of a subject-subject or subject-object relationship may be used as a measure when analyzing communication situations. At this moment, are we giving all those present every possibility to access the information being given? Is every person in this communication situation able to make use of his or her natural abilities? If the answer is yes, then we have created a subject-subject relationship based on the principles of freedom of speech. The participants are equal partners and have the same chance to form an opinion. If the answer is no, then we have created a subject-object relationship where some of the people present do not have the same access to the information as others. Subject-subject relationships are part of the communication setting in which all participants have information in common; they are collective and enable everyone to understand what is being communicated.

CONCLUDING REMARKS

Cochlear implants have been represented by researchers in the media as having created a totally new situation: babies who are implanted and who receive an oral education are expected to become almost hearing (see Komesaroff, this volume). Deaf people's experience is generally ignored and considered irrelevant to this new generation of cochlear implanted children. Viewing Deaf people's stories as representing only the past devalues their knowledge and rejects their life experience. And no one can be sure that the children being operated on so early in life will become "almost hearing." We are therefore experiencing a vacuum in which the arguments made by each side are rejected by the other as each waits for the "evidence" to come—perhaps in two years, four years, or ten years. I introduced this chapter by suggesting that the controversy over oralism and sign language may be represented as a spiral rather than as the traditional notion of a pendulum swinging in one direction and then the other. As we add the issue of childhood implantation to the controversy, it seems that we are unsure where to move within the spiral.

The Deaf community is now more open and accepting of implant recipients than it was some years ago (described, for example, in Christiansen and Leigh 2002). The atmosphere of skepticism that persisted for some years in relation to the operation has changed to concern about what happens to these children after the operation takes place. At the same time, native sign languages are finally being accepted all around the world after the language and culture of Deaf communities has been suppressed for almost 200 years (Austria, Belgium, and New Zealand Sign Languages are the latest to have been recognized by their country's respective parliaments). But the arguments being made by some cochlear implant supporters are not conducive to gaining the support of the Deaf community: negative views on the use of sign language, reports of "salvation," the supposed ignorance of deaf people and their experience, claims of economic benefit, and representations of "normality."

First, suggesting that sign language *not* be used in the education of deaf children with cochlear implants (which accounts for most of the new generation of young people) ignores and devalues deaf and hard of hearing people's experience. Technological development cannot (and perhaps should not) be stopped. But deaf people have struggled to make the hearing community aware that a person is more than his or her ears: quality of life cannot be measured in decibels. Language and identity are so closely connected that having one's language devalued subsequently devalues one's being and puts that person—in this case, deaf people—into an "object" position. An attack on one's mother tongue is an attack on one's identity. When some people say that sign language should not be used with children who have cochlear implants, many deaf people remember when they were young and struggled to understand their teachers through speechreading. They empathize with those deaf children today who have cochlear implants. Until sign language is fully accepted, many deaf people feel they still have to fight for the rights of deaf children.

Second, media accounts of cochlear implants as a "salvation" for deaf children are simplified and sensationalized, and they misrepresent the richness of deaf people's lives. I admit I can understand that it is exciting for people who do not know anything about deafness to read that deafness has been "cured." If I read a headline, "Blind child can now see," I too may forget that this claim is a simplified truth, and I might start praising the doctors.

Third, some medical professionals and the associations they represent show an unwillingness to meet with Deaf people and listen to their experience. Those who fight for a purely oral means of communication for deaf children with implants may think that cochlear implantation is so revolutionary that deaf people today have nothing to offer a child who has been implanted as a one-year-old. Such views will be met with resistance from Deaf people.

Fourth, the financial argument sometimes used by oralists who state that the community will benefit economically when deaf children have been implanted is offensive to many Deaf people. The suggestion is that the cost of sign language interpreters and schools for deaf students will decrease. Whether or not such arguments are valid on some level, Deaf people are offended when their lives and education are considered primarily as an expense for the society as a whole.

Finally, where does the representation of the ability to hear as being "normal" leave Deaf people? The media make announcements that, through cochlear implants, Deaf children can have a normal life. This view of normality is exclusionary and reductionist because it includes only certain members of the society. Deafness is present in all societies and, thus, is one of the characteristics that makes up a diverse community. It is not acceptable for the dominant group in a society to impose a particular view of reality on all its members. The definition of normal, rather than be narrowed to include only some members of society, should be expanded to include those who have made a variety of choices (such as using sign language), even if other members of the society may not understand.

As Deaf adults, we can identify with the parents' circumstances; we meet them and show our understanding that having a deaf child can be a shock for them. When medical professionals, more often now than in the past, recommend a purely oral education, we have to be patient and try to argue for the addition of sign language. But if we argue without thinking of the other person's feelings, then we are trying to persuade rather than convince. In this way, we make ourselves the subject and the other the object, and we get caught up in the subject-object trap. We need to inform doctors, teachers, and parents so they understand that deaf children can profit from sign language. It may take a long time, but we must never give up fighting for what we believe in. For deaf people—with or without cochlear implants, with or without residual hearing—every opportunity must be taken to create a subject-subject relationship to ensure their freedom of speech.

REFERENCES

Bateman, G. C. 1996. Attitudes of the Deaf community toward political activism. In *Cultural and language diversity and the Deaf experience*, ed. I. Parasnis, 160–71. New York: Cambridge University Press.

Bjørndal, P. S. 1981. *Fra Lille Bloksbjerg til Nedre Gausen skole* [From little Bloksbjerg to Nedre Gausen School]. Holmestrand, Norway: Nedre Gausen Resource Centre.

Christiansen, J. B., and I. Leigh. 2002. *Cochlear implants in children: Ethics and choices.* Washington, D.C.: Gallaudet University Press.

Peterson, P. R. 2001. Døv identitet og politisk deltakelse [Deaf identify and political participation]. Unpublished thesis, Department of Political Science, University of Oslo, Norway.

———. 2004. Political participation among deaf people. Paper presented at the 2nd International Deaf Academics and Researchers Conference, February 19–21, Gallaudet University, Washington, D.C.

———. 2005. *Tegnspråkopplæring er det beste som kunne hendt oss!* [Sign language training is the best thing that could have hapened to us!]. Holmestrand, Norway: Nedre Gausen Resource Centre and Landsdekkende Informasions og Koordineringsutvalg for Tegnspråkopplaeringen for Foreldre.

Skjervheim, H. B. 1968. *Det liberale dilemma og andre essays* [The liberal dilemma and other essays]. Oslo, Norway: Tanum.

United Nations (UN). 1948. *Universal declaration of human rights,* General Assembly resolution 217 A [III], 10 December.

10

DEAF AUSTRALIANS AND THE COCHLEAR IMPLANT: REPORTING FROM GROUND LEVEL

Karen Lloyd and Michael Uniacke

I read a great many of the books on deafness and the deaf—all of them by non-deaf specialists—and ended up feeling considerably deafer than when I started. A minimal but frequent condescension of attitude and tone left me with a slightly depressed ego.

—David Wright (1969, 201)

The English poet David Wright was one of an exceedingly rare species—a deaf person who has had published an account of what it is like to be deaf. In the quote above, Wright was explaining his choice to write about deafness before starting to read about it. He wrote those words during the 1960s, well before the cochlear implant or digital technology was to make its impact. The world has changed a great deal since then, but not everything has changed. We know very well Wright's feeling from the "non-deaf specialists." We would say the "condescension of attitude and tone" is worse—much worse now than in the 1960s—and it is largely because of the cochlear implant debate.

The combined experience of this chapter's authors, that of mixing with the Deaf community and with other deaf and hard of hearing people in Australia, in all their shapes and colors, totals more than sixty years. As Deaf people, we have participated in paid and in voluntary capacities as writers, as researchers, and as contributors in other roles. Our involvement includes participation in state and national organizations of Deaf people, welfare organizations, self-help groups, and hard of hearing groups. We have associated with parents, with teachers, with welfare workers, and with interpreters. We knew the Deaf community before the cochlear implant was well known, and we have observed and written about the community's early responses to it. We have observed the way in which the cochlear implant debate threatened to become a major battleground between Deaf and hearing people. We have watched the twists and turns in the debate as the early anger from Deaf people diluted into an easy acceptance of those Deaf people with cochlear implants who began to surface within this community. What did remain consistent were the occasional spikes of arrogance from medical specialists against Deaf people, to an extent that would make David Wright blush. Yet Deaf Australians have done what they usually have done. They simply get on with living, which is, we think, the best possible response they could have given.

In this chapter, we report on the cochlear implant debate in its Australian context (Australia was the country where the multichannel cochlear implant was developed and made commercially available through the work of Professor Graeme Clark at the University of Melbourne). Our report comes from our decades of combined experiences, from the personal, from the political, and from being part of the community of Deaf people in Australia.

Where Did It Start?

We do not know where the debate about the cochlear implant started. We had always known there was research into cures for deafness. We hoped it would help those deaf people who wanted a cure.

> *Karen:*[1] My mother, years ago, persuaded me to go talk to an audiologist about the possibility of a cochlear implant, before it became well known. I fought her on it but eventually gave in to her. The audiologist agreed that, for me, it would be a waste of time, effort, and money.
>
> * * *
>
> *Michael:* My first indication of the debate came from fundraising appeals on television during the 1970s. They were called telethons and were conducted for sixteen- and seventeen-hour stretches. They were designed to raise funds for research into nerve deafness. I remembered feeling very uneasy about these telethons. I was discovering deafness, and deaf people, and these telethons amounted to very considerable publicity. I was part of a group of deaf people. We had something to say about being deaf, and the telethons might have been a good way for us to tell the world. But the hearing people who controlled it were profoundly uninterested in us and in anything we might have wanted to say.

As the cochlear implant became better known, the Deaf community was aghast. Hearing people stirred up a great deal of "fear and loathing" within the Deaf community. They made statements about how the cochlear implant was going to eradicate the Deaf community. The media was reporting this new miracle cure for deafness. In Victoria, the southernmost state of mainland Australia, the annual telethons continued to raise funds for cochlear implant research, and their message about deaf people worsened. They promoted the cochlear implant by portraying deaf people as deprived, helpless, and doomed to live in a world of silence unless viewers donated money to help a cure called the bionic ear. They showed deaf children begging viewers for money to help those who were deaf. In 1986, Peter Howson, the former Liberal (conservative party) member of the house of representatives and ex-chairman of the Victorian Deafness Foundation, declared in a speech at the Annual General Meeting of the Victorian School for Deaf Children (September 22, 1986) that as a result of cochlear implants and other technological developments, in forty years' time, there may well not be an adult Deaf community in Victoria as we then knew it.

Such pronouncements caused great consternation in the Deaf community. Who was this man? What would he know about the Deaf community? Had he ever spoken to any of us? Did he try to find out what we thought of all these developments? How could he say our community would die out? What would Deaf people do without their Deaf community? It was unimaginable, a terrifying scenario to contemplate.

But at the same time, there was good news. The Deaf community in Australia was beginning to learn more about itself. The term "Auslan" was coined as a name for the sign language used in the community, and Auslan was included in discussions about an Australian languages policy. Auslan was officially recognized as a community language by the Australian Government (see Lo Bianco 1987), and Deaf people began to talk about their sign language as a language.

Until then, hearing educators had led Deaf people to believe that their language was just an easy way for them to communicate. Deaf people were taught that signs were impoverished, were mere gestures, were not a real language like English, and were the reason for their difficulty in acquiring English literacy. To then have linguists now showing Deaf people that their sign language was in fact a real language was to many of us incredible and deeply empowering.

> *Karen:* In the late 1980s, Breda Carty, a Deaf teacher of deaf students, began holding "Deaf Studies" workshops for the community, and many of us went along to learn more about ourselves, our history, and our community, both worldwide and within Australia. These workshops were enthralling for Deaf people. I remember being in the audience at a conference when Carty made her first presentation about Deaf history. It was at this conference that she recounted Lane's (1984) chronicle of Jean-Marc Itard, a French doctor who in the early nineteenth century attempted a variety of cures for deafness on the pupils of the deaf school in Paris:
>
>> Itard tried fracturing the skull of a few pupils, striking the area just behind the ear with a hammer. With a dozen pupils he applied a white-hot metal button behind the ear, which led to pus and a scab in about a week. Yet another of Itard's treatments was to thread a string through a pupil's neck with a seton needle, which caused a suppurating wound that supposedly allowed "feculent humours" to dry up. In addition, several of the pupils in the school were badly scarred from his use of the moxa, an old Chinese remedy. (Lane 1984, 134)
>
> I remember the powerful reactions of the mostly Deaf audience, who looked around at each other, shocked and appalled. Some became very upset and cried. Some laughed incredulously. But the most common reaction was cynical. "What's changed?" people said. "Now we have the cochlear implant!"

Deaf Studies and the recognition of Auslan as a language to be respected brought a new strength to the Deaf community. A better knowledge of ourselves, our history, our language, our community and its endurance through the ages, as well as its ability to withstand attacks on it, brought a new vitality. The Australian Association of the Deaf (AAD) was formed in 1986, and gathered momentum in the late 1980s and early 1990s. There was a stronger feeling of certainty and a braver sense of having the right to speak out for ourselves, to openly disagree with "the experts." And the Deaf community did fight back against the attitudes promoted by the cochlear implant. We wrote letters to the doctors who were trashing our community and our language. We wrote to the media who wrote about us as if we were all desperately seeking a cure from this wretched silent world in which we were supposed to be wallowing. We published articles in newsletters and magazines. We made speeches at conferences.

Karen: The AAD adopted a policy on the cochlear implant, calling for a moratorium on the use of the cochlear implant in children. During an interview on national television, the then AAD president, Colin Allen, made a comment about facial paralysis in cochlear implant operations, which upset one of the implant centers. The center wrote to the AAD and threatened legal action. I remember this vividly because, at the time, I was secretary of the AAD. I remember Allen showing me this letter and the look of alarm on his face. I laughed and said, "They're bluffing. They think you are just a dumb deaf person who can be intimidated. We will get legal advice and call their bluff." Eventually, after an exchange of letters between lawyers, the matter was dropped.

* * *

Michael: I remember a physical reaction when I read in the Melbourne newspaper *The Age* about the news of a grant made to the cochlear implant research program from the United States (Menagh 1987, 1). The grant was made by the director of a U.S. prosthetics program and was for $1.75 million. In that article, the director, Dr. Terry Hambrecht, claimed the purpose of the cochlear implant was "to eradicate deafness, in the same way that diseases like smallpox had been controlled."

I was appalled and I was seething. I spent much of that day composing a letter to the paper, a letter I knew I would never send. Venting in this letter was how I coped with being told that a part of myself, part of a core of who I was, was something abhorrent and disgusting.

The worst part of the way in which the cochlear implant fueled attacks on Deaf people and the Deaf community was not the cochlear implant itself. The worse part was the banal arrogance of the men and women who pronounced those attacks. It was as though we were bugs and they trod all over us. The cochlear implant was drawing support from people who knew nothing about Deaf people. The more that various hearing people thought they knew best, the more they were upset by Deaf people who protested. Perhaps they were upset because the protests enabled the wider community to gain glimpses of insight that they understood that the audiological version of *Father Knows Best* might not leave everyone hearing happily ever after.

The Deaf community knew, and has always known, what it is like to be deaf. Deaf people knew very well that there are good things and bad things about being deaf. It rarely occurred to hearing people to ask Deaf people. That being ignored was the sticking point. Information was needed for parents who discovered they had a deaf child, and none of this information came from the people who knew about it better than anyone else—better than teachers, social workers, doctors, and scientists. And Deaf people found that they were expected to be joyfully anticipating a "cure" while their language and community was being ignored.

TECHNOLOGICAL VERSION OF *FATHER KNOWS BEST*

The cochlear implant is the latest of a long list of technology developed by hearing professionals whose mission in life is to cure the sick and rehabilitate the impaired.

When we were children, box hearing aids were the most common. Then hearing aids were progressively improved and became more powerful. Now we have cochlear implants, the most powerful of all to date and continually being improved.

> *Karen:* In all the years that I have been an advocate, I have heard the counter-argument from "professionals" again and again that goes along the lines of "but your experience is not valid anymore because technology has improved and is more powerful and successful now. It can do so much more than it could in your day." It is a powerful argument for silencing the Deaf dissenting view, and it is potent when presented to parents.

The advances-of-technology argument falls flat the moment we realize that Deaf people acquire more powerful and sophisticated hearing aids, yet still remain part of the Deaf community, and when we realize that Deaf people with cochlear implants are doing just the same. The situation is identical to that within the numerous centers for hard of hearing people around the country whose members likewise acquire and use the latest technology, but do not necessarily leave their community of the hard of hearing. Both Deaf and hard of hearing people stick together for a reason that is unbelievably simple.

If there is such a marvel as a god of technology in the twenty-first century, it is as proud and possessive as the emblematic nineteenth-century jealous queen who ruled the kingdom of speech. The Reverend Giulio Tarra promoted this queen[2] at the 1880 Congress of Milan, which decided to abolish the world's sign languages in favor of speech in the education of deaf children around the world. The cochlear implant is merely the latest of more than 120 years of attempts to eliminate deafness, and by implication, the Deaf community. Nothing really has changed.

Do As I Say, Not As I Communicate

> *Michael:* The concern of hearing people that Deaf people be enabled to hear is contradicted by the way in which some hearing professionals speak to Deaf people. Once, in the company of a hearing colleague, I visited a major educational and early-intervention center for deaf children. This center subscribed strongly to the view that speech training and early fitting of hearing aids or a cochlear implant were essential for the deaf child to function "in a hearing world." Sign language was not necessary. I visited in good faith, to learn what they do and to see their facilities. I was treated with courtesy. I had two impressions. One was of the facilities—a bright and spacious center with friendly staff members, in a lovely setting.
>
> My other impression was of amazement. The senior staff member who showed us around knew very well that I was Deaf. It did not change her communication habits. She made very little eye contact with me. She preferred to look at my hearing colleague. At times, I had to interject comments to remind her that I was there—and to make me feel less like I was unimportant and inconsequential. Incredibly, she would speak to us as we followed her along corridors and across rooms, leaving me to attempt to lipread the back

of her head. I pointed out this situation to her; I said I was Deaf and I needed to see her face when she spoke. Of course she was apologetic; most people are. But she continued to forget this basic rule of communication decorum. This woman, who was supposed to be an expert in deaf education, had no idea how to communicate with Deaf adults.

* * *

Karen: Michael's experience (above) is not unusual. I have had similar experiences with many teachers of deaf students and other "experts" who work with deaf children, for example, speech pathologists and other therapists. There are the teachers who are hard to speechread or who use signed English. But I do not really know signed English; I use Auslan. Signed English is used in Australian schools by hearing teachers of deaf students, but it is not widely used in the Deaf community. It is very different from Auslan; it is awkward, even painful to use and watch, and it is not visually logical. Teachers who use Signed English become impatient when I do not understand. And there are the teachers who have no experience with interpreters. During a meeting with a group of teachers of deaf students, another Deaf person, and an interpreter, the teachers had no idea how to work with the interpreter—nor did they have any idea of such basic rules as only one person should talk at a time. At the policy and service review meetings I have attended with teachers and therapists, only those who can sign make any attempt to communicate with me during the breaks, and the oralist experts form separate huddles of their own.

Both of us speak, lipread, and use Auslan. Both of us are good at all three. Both of us associate freely with Deaf and hearing people in our everyday lives. Why are some deafness "experts" so difficult for us to communicate with?

OH MY GOD, MY CHILD IS DEAF

Parents want the best for their children. So, how do they work out what is best for their child? When parents are hearing and have no previous knowledge of deafness, this challenge is the major issue. Where do they go to get factual, accurate, realistic information?

As advocates, we always want to know, what is the quality of the information that the parents are given at the time of diagnosis? We have listened to parents who have complained about being railroaded into a cochlear implant for their child, right at the moment when their child's deafness has been confirmed.

Likewise, what is the quality of information about deafness that is taught to teachers of deaf students? What are they told about the cochlear implant? What are they told about deafness? Do the teachers know any Deaf adults personally—not as children, not as clients, not as former pupils nor as special cases, but as friends and equals? And we also need to ask, where did those teachers' information on deafness come from? In the early 1990s, the major university that was training teachers of the deaf in Melbourne devoted one hour from the one-year course to provide instruction about the Deaf community, thus ensuring that teachers knew little more than that the Deaf community existed and that Auslan was its language.

> *Karen:* In 2004, I gave a presentation at a parents' conference in Sydney. I commented on the way cochlear implant clinics for children do not give parents accurate information about the Deaf community and Auslan. During the ensuing discussion, a therapist from a cochlear implant clinic said they do give information to the parents, and they do not try to force the cochlear implant on them. A hearing parent of a deaf child then said that this claim was not true. She said she had been to this same therapist's clinic. The staff members had told her she was a cruel mother because she had chosen not to have her deaf child implanted.

What do parents go through? First, the child's deafness is diagnosed by health professionals and audiologists. These are the hearing people whose mission in life is supposedly to cure the sick and rehabilitate the impaired. These are the people who give the parents their first advice. They regard the child's deafness as something "wrong" that needs to be "fixed" so that the child can be "normal." The cochlear implant is now included in this early information and advice to parents about their options. It is presented very early as a solution to this "problem" and gives the parents hope where, until then, all seemed grim and hopeless, no doubt. Now, with universal hearing screening for newborn babies, the cochlear implant option is being presented almost the moment the child is born.

> *Karen:* I have met so many parents who say that either (a) nobody told them about the Deaf community and Auslan or (b) they were advised not to allow the child to sign or mix with deaf people who sign. I have often wondered why so few parents contact organizations such as the Australian Association of the Deaf—organizations that can give them accurate information about the Deaf community and Auslan and that can introduce them to Deaf adults who are living independent, successful, fulfilling lives.
>
> Over the years, I have listened to educational professionals say to me, "but it's the parents who make the decisions." I have listened to parents who say, "but this is what the teachers or professionals advised me." I have watched parents take government education departments to court in an effort to have their children gain access to the type of educational programs the parents believed were best for their child. All the while, educational professionals were claiming "but it's the parents who decide what type of education they want."

What happens is that the educators decide to provide certain programs, and the parents must choose between them. If the parents want something different for their children, for example, access to an education through the language used by Deaf people, then they have to fight very hard for it. Some are defeated by the system, some have won, and—after the education authorities have appealed the decision—have won again (see Komesaroff 2006).

If parents had ready access to information about deafness and the abilities and potential of Deaf people, they would quite possibly have a different attitude. The most authentic information about deafness comes from Deaf people themselves, and it is very difficult to obtain access to books, films, artwork, or other forms of creative expression that give the Deaf point of view. It is easy, however, to find stories about overcoming deafness (see Ackehurst 2000).

DEAF KIDS, THEIR HEARING PARENTS, AND OURS

Almost every deaf person we know with hearing parents—and that has been the vast majority of them—has had a problematic relationship with his or her parents. Problems have ranged from early battles about wearing hearing aids to insinuations from parents that mixing with other deaf kids is a mark of failure. Most Deaf people eventually grow beyond these battles and come to terms with their parents. Most begin to understand and appreciate the ways in which their parents were grappling not only with their own sense of bewilderment but also with misleading, contradictory, and sometimes offensive advice given to them by hearing professionals. But for some Deaf people, there is life-long estrangement from their hearing parents.

There are many deaf people who have come to the Deaf community in their late teens or early twenties. They have lived a life trying to fit in with the so-called hearing world and trying to be the kind of "normal" person their parents hope they will be. Many of these young Deaf people are angry—with their parents, with hearing people in general. But is it really the parents who are at fault?

Karen: My mother told me the story of the very first advice she received from a doctor when I became deaf at eight years old in the 1960s: "Put her in an institution and forget about her." Later, a professional said I needed to go to the specialist deaf school and be with other deaf children; if she did not send me there, she was putting me at a disadvantage. Yet another professional told my mother that if she did send me to a deaf school, she would be putting me at a disadvantage.

My mother told me recently, "how was I to know which of this professional advice was in your best interests?" Forty years later, this situation still happens.

* * *

Michael: One medical specialist told my parents that one of my older deaf sisters was mentally retarded. My parents were also told that a brief "ray" treatment "to pierce a blockage" would cure deafness. My father physically intervened when another specialist believed it was appropriate to impose pain on my sister during a hearing test. My parents did not want to have anything to do with what my father called "special social workers." They did not want to have anything to do with deaf schools. My mother once told me they would rather see me at the bottom of a class of hearing kids than at the top of a class of deaf kids. That view was their way of saying that deaf schools would not challenge us enough; deaf schools' standards and expectations of deaf kids were very low. I do not know where they got this impression of standards at deaf schools. It was a theme repeated to me many times by teachers—the low expectations. No one seriously expected that deaf kids would achieve. My mother told me many times, "It was unheard of for hard of hearing children to get to secondary school."

* * *

Karen: When I was eleven, I took off my hearing aid and put it away in a drawer. My mother took it out one day and suggested I wear it. I refused. My mother asked why. "The teachers said it will help you lipread," she said.

But I was adamant. "It doesn't help me lipread, it makes it harder," I said. "It is too hard to try and work out what I'm hearing and, at the same time, put together what I'm seeing. It is easier to lipread without it." My mother looked at me thoughtfully, and put the hearing aid back in the drawer.

Years later, I asked her, "Why did you listen to me and not to the advice you were given by the experts?"

"There were many reasons," she replied, "but in the end, I believed that you were old enough and smart enough to know what you were talking about. If you did get something worthwhile from a hearing aid, you would not have refused to wear it."

These "experts" also told my mother I should never learn to sign because I would become lazy and forget how to talk. Years later when I did learn to sign (and could still remember how to speak), my mother asked, would it help if she also learned?

* * *

Michael: My parents had no exposure to sign language. They knew nothing about the Deaf community other than that deaf children were not educated beyond the basics and were capable only of menial employment. They discouraged their deaf children from associating with other deaf people.

Decades later, my mother made the astonishing admission that perhaps the attitudes of her and my father were wrong. She thought, perhaps they should have allowed me to mix with other hard of hearing children. She even said that perhaps she and my father should have made some attempt to learn sign language.

"It was obvious to Dad and I how much happier you had become when you started going around with that crowd of hard of hearing young people," she told me. "You had made up your own mind by then."

I said to her, no, it was not a question of whether their attitudes were right or wrong. The answer was that they did their best with what they knew. And what they knew of deafness was that their children were far more capable than what the experts told them. More recently, my mother accompanied one of her daughters who took one of her grandsons for a hearing test. "And nothing has changed," she told me. "After all these years, these fellows who are supposed to know all about the hard of hearing, still don't know anything."

* * *

Karen: I have met parents of deaf children who are now grown up. They have told me that they wished they had known then what they know now. In the twenty years I have been an advocate for Deaf people's rights, I have observed repeated waves of parents receiving the same type of information from the experts. It is best for the child to learn to speak and "be normal," they said. Children should not learn to sign, and it is best that they not be with other deaf children, especially deaf children who sign, they added. Then the child grows up and joins the Deaf community and learns to sign—and blossoms. The parents wonder about the advice they were given way back then. It happens over and over again. Parents are not being given opportunities to learn from the experiences of other parents, and they are not learning from Deaf people themselves.

* * *

Michael: It is a pity that it is easier to remember the worst experiences. In my time at the then Victorian Deaf Society, I remember a father who refused to allow his teenage deaf daughter to use public transport. Another set of parents treated their middle-aged son like a schoolboy. He was not allowed to do anything without their permission. I'm sure others have similar stories. It is sad and depressing.

I remember, too, some of the uproar with the deaf group Earforce during the 1980s. Earforce was an independent group run by Deaf people. They started a deaf youth group run by older Deaf people. Some parents of the younger deaf people had problems understanding that Deaf people could make capable youth leaders. Some parents were on the lookout for the slightest sign of trouble, the merest hint that things were not going well, as "proof" that Deaf people generally were incapable of many things. They were concerned that one of them was looking after young deaf people. To varying degrees, the views of some teachers reflected this attitude.

The saddest thing, from my point of view, is the way deaf kids absorb the attitude from their parents that hearing is good and deafness is bad. They regard things deaf as "beneath" them, and they are quick to assume the worst about Deaf people.

We know many oral deaf kids have this attitude when they first come to the Deaf community. They see themselves as superior to Deaf people who sign. They feel that way because they have had it drummed into them that they must not sign, that it is better to speak and be like hearing people, that signing is a "fallback" position for people who cannot cope in the "hearing world," that signing is only for "failures." Over time, many change their views and attitudes as they meet and mix more with Deaf people who sign. So often, they become more self-confident, and develop new skills that they then take with them into their jobs and activities in hearing-dominated environments.

However, there are many deaf people in the Deaf community who have grown up oral and have been, and remain, damaged. Common examples of this damage are Deaf people who are angry and very antihearing as well as Deaf people who need constant attention and reassurance that they are "good enough" or are doing well. They have grown up with this type of attention.

Karen: In my experience, the most well-adjusted Deaf people are often those who come from Deaf families; often, they also are among the most well-educated, have better general knowledge, and have a better understanding of the wider world around them. Among the "converts"—deaf people who have been brought up orally and who later join the Deaf community and learn Auslan—we find, when we dig deep enough, that many of those with a better educational level and general knowledge actually became deaf in mid-childhood or late childhood. In other words, they became deaf after acquiring fluent language and some education.

* * *

Michael: I have had some marvelous discussions with parents. I know why we get on so well. It is because in us they see a glimpse of the future for their deaf daughters and their deaf sons. They are extremely interested when I talk about what happened to me at the same stage of life as their sons. Again, these parents leave themselves open to new attitudes. They have a willingness to explore. We give them information and insights that no hearing specialist can give them.

DEAF ADOLESCENTS

We are unabatedly interested in the attitudes of deaf adolescents. Adolescence is about asking who you are, what your place is in the world. For deaf teens, the question becomes, Am I Deaf or am I hearing? Their parents want them to be "hearing." But it is easier for these teens to communicate with deaf peers. Those with cochlear implants who choose the Deaf path are almost saying to their parents, you were wrong. Of course, the reality is never as simple as that, but that message lurks under the surface.

Deaf people, sooner or later, but probably most often during adolescence, need to reconcile the Deaf and hearing aspects of themselves. If a deaf person has been brought up within the hearing community and has had little or no contact with the Deaf community, then this reconciliation is likely to be more difficult and he or she may experience more disruption in various relationships. This disruption can, and often does, damage the person's relationships with family, but most deaf people eventually do work out some kind of truce. Most people who are part of the Deaf community live bilingual and bicultural lives to varying degrees. Parents often do not seem to understand this need for deaf children to go through this process of discovering their Deaf self and reconciling the Deaf and hearing selves. After all, who ever really explains this need to parents?

Cochlear implant programs show a significant lack of interest in what happens to deaf children when they hit adolescence. Those programs seem interested only in children. Professor Graeme Clark's (2000) book, *Sounds from Silence*, has a cover dominated by images of small children. There is a staggering lack of research into the attitudes of the children with cochlear implants who reach adolescence.

We planned to interview young deaf people who had received a cochlear implant as a child. We wanted to record their stories, in their own words. We wanted to hear the whole range of views—from those whose cochlear implant has worked well, from those for whom the cochlear implant failed, and from those whose experience has been in between.

We talked with people we know who have a cochlear implant. We talked with people who have direct contact with not only people who have a cochlear implant but also their families. We produced a letter for distribution, telling of our plans. But no one wanted to be interviewed. Of two people we contacted directly ourselves, one (whose experience of the cochlear implant has, we believe, been positive) did not reply. The other, whose experience has been negative and who no longer uses her cochlear implant, declined to participate. She did not want to discuss her experiences. An intermediary suggested that this second person did not wish to speak out publicly because she did not wish to upset her parents.

One of our contacts personally approached two potential interviewees and asked them directly whether they would like to be involved, but both declined. One apparently wanted to be seen as a person, as her own self—distinct from someone with a cochlear implant.

This reluctance to be interviewed is intriguing to us. Why does no one want to talk about their experiences with the cochlear implant? We thought it would be difficult to find people who would be prepared to say anything negative about their cochlear implant. We thought this way for a number of reasons but mainly because so much is invested in cochlear implants in terms of time, money, hard work, emotions, hopes, and dreams, and we expected people to be reluctant to say anything that might upset their parents, given how much parents invest in the cochlear implant. We also were aware that many adolescents and young adults have not yet worked out for themselves what they really think and feel about many things.

Karen: Apart from one year at a specialized school for the deaf when I was ten, I spent my formative years surrounded by hearing people, and I never met another deaf person until I was eighteen and at university. I grew up believing that signing was bad and that it was bad to mix with other deaf people, who were inferior to me because they signed. I was a classic oral snob. I believed those things because they were what I had been taught. When I was in year 11 at school, a family friend who was training to be a teacher asked me to speak about my experiences at one of her college tutorials. I went along and talked about how good my teachers were at including me, and it was garbage. I was saying what I thought I was supposed to say. I was saying what I needed to say to be accepted and to be thought of as a good girl.

Then I became involved as a volunteer with a school for deaf students. It was an oral school and it did not take me long to realize the kids were not learning, they were not communicating, and I could not communicate with them. That was when I started to rethink all the things I thought I believed. I worked out what I really thought and believed, as distinct from what other (hearing) people had told me to think and believe. And that was when I decided I wanted to meet other Deaf adults and learn to sign. That was the beginning of my own personal journey of discovering my Deaf self.

I think this sort of experience is common with young people, it takes time for many of us to break away and become brave and confident enough to say what we really think. So I think that it will be some time yet before we will readily find Deaf people with cochlear implants who are ready to say what they really think and feel as distinct from what other people want them to think and feel.

What we are seeing now is youths with cochlear implants appearing at the door of the Deaf community. We are opening up that door and saying, oh alright, come in. The Deaf community still has some ambivalence, but young deaf people with cochlear implants are not being rejected.

We think much of this ambivalence that the Deaf community has toward oral deaf people and people with cochlear implants arises not so much because of their ability to speak or because of the cochlear implant in itself. The ambivalence arises because the "immigrants" bring with them an attitude, bred in them by the attitudes of hearing people around them, that speech and listening is superior to sign language and that they are therefore superior to Deaf people who use Auslan. It takes time for the Deaf community to knock this attitude out of them, and while Deaf people are doing this purging, they have to suffer the attitude. So we think that this ambivalence is understandable. Cochlear implant devotees, however, take this ambivalence and try to turn it into something that is not necessarily so—into hostility toward people with cochlear implants just because they have a cochlear implant.

If a person with a cochlear implant comes into the Deaf community and is respectful toward Auslan and the Deaf community, then the cochlear implant is scarcely an issue. The key to the Deaf community's attitude is not the cochlear implant but attitudes about Auslan and Deaf people.

The AAD policy on the cochlear implant was revised and was adopted by AAD members at its General Meeting on November 3, 2006. This updated version includes information about the need for children with cochlear implants to still have access to Auslan and the Deaf community; those children are still deaf children, and they still need to be respected as deaf children, not as "broken hearing children who need to be fixed." The cochlear implant essentially does not change any of the age-old issues with which deaf children have had to grapple.

BUT I WANT TO HEAR AGAIN

Michael: Of my numerous freelance writing assignments, one that I like the most is my 1987 article on the cochlear implant (Uniacke 1987). This article was the first in Australia to ask Deaf people themselves what they thought about the cochlear implant. I was not at all surprised to learn that it attracted mail from hearing impaired people who were appalled that anyone could have any kind of opinion on the cochlear implant other than unqualified praise. The letters, which were brought to my attention too late for a reply, were published in 1988 in a magazine by Self Help for the Hard of Hearing, which also republished the article without my knowledge.

I recalled thinking that all but one of those letters indicated how strongly many people desired to regain a sensation of hearing. Who could have a problem with that? Their responses impressed on me the diversity of people with hearing loss and how careful we needed to be when we spoke about deaf people.

The one letter that interested me above all the others came from a woman named Margaret Haenke (1988, 11), who was prominent in the leadership of this organization. She demanded to know of me: "Has he bothered to learn to speak?" The chain of logic leading to this question gave me some enjoyable hours of speculation. It seemed to go like this:

- All deaf people want to be able to hear.
- The wonderful cochlear implant enables us to hear.
- If we are now able to hear, we are now able to speak.
- We all live in a hearing world where everyone speaks.
- Therefore all deaf people have a chance to better themselves.
- Michael's appalling article reveals people who cannot be bothered to better themselves.
- Therefore it could only have been written by someone who can neither hear nor speak.

Part of my fantasy, of course, was constructing a reply. Included in my reply would be a tape of a broadcast in which I was interviewed a few years earlier for a radio feature on the International Year of Disabled People. I would have added another tape of a broadcast I did for a book review for the Australian Broadcasting Commission's *Science Show*. And the sweetest touch on this delicious irony? The book was about American Sign Language.

But the main purpose of any reply was not to point out that I could speak. It was to reveal the entrenched, hardline, and undeviating attitudes in a black-and-white view of the cochlear implant. This black-and-white view produced absurd leaps in logic and a profound failure to comprehend the considerable diversity of attitudes within and about deafness and what it means.

It is easy to understand the frustration of people who describe themselves as hearing impaired. Their use of the word *hearing* in what they call themselves suggests they dearly wish to regain a sense of something they remembered and had lost. This wish is the common theme in their repeated descriptions of what their experience is like with a cochlear implant that works, and their descriptions are indeed most joyful. We would struggle to think of anyone who would deny them this opportunity to regain a sensation of hearing. But we part company with hearing impaired people when they promote attitudes that insist deaf people are deficient and the cochlear implant will make us whole again.

DID ANYBODY EVER ASK US?

We struggle to recall any instance when any health or medical professional has ever approached any organization run by Deaf people themselves and asked for information about Auslan or the Deaf community. Professionals are supposed to be well-informed in their field. But apparently very few have considered the views of the very people they purport to help.

When hearing people actually seek the views of deaf people, it is extremely unusual. Harlan Lane (1984, 63) gave one example from the 1760s, involving the founder of deaf education, the abbé de l'Epée:

Still, it was the abbé de l'Epée, son of the king's architect, who first turned to the poor, despised, illiterate deaf and said, "Teach Me." And this act of humility gained him everlasting glory. It is his true title to our gratitude, for in becoming the student of his pupils, in seeking to learn their signs, he equipped himself to educate them and to found the education of the deaf.

The cochlear implant program in Melbourne was established in 1970. We are not aware of any attempt it made to inform Deaf people until 1988.[3] That was when Deaf people themselves—the AAD's Victorian Council of Deaf People—organized a forum and invited a representative from the program.

If the program itself bothered very little with the views of the Deaf community, its corporate arm, Cochlear Ltd., bothers not at all. Cochlear Ltd.'s CEOs bemoan the fact that many more deaf people could be implanted than have actually taken up the technology. The company's former CEO, Jack O'Mahoney (cited in Pheasant 2003), had these comments to make about those without a cochlear implant:

"Look at the alternative if they didn't have (a cochlear implant)," he says. "How selective is their employment? How specific is their schooling, how difficult is their family life because everyone has to try to cater for this person?" . . . Rather than being a burden, an implant recipient becomes a productive member of society. "It is so significant a solution that you are immediately going to get a taxpayer again instead of a tax dependant, and you are restoring a quality of life that was previously unavailable," he says.

This view of Deaf people asserts that in social, economic, and employment terms, they are useless, but a cochlear implant will restore them. This claim being the case, a cochlear implant will also benefit a great many hearing people.

But according to Professor Bill Gibson, a Sydney cochlear implant surgeon and supporter, Deaf people are doomed anyway. Quoted in Stephens (1994), he has reasoned that "by 2000, no child will be handicapped by deafness." This development will be just as well, he asserts elsewhere, because "Deaf adults have limited social and job opportunities. 60 per cent of adults who can communicate only by using sign are either unemployed or under employed" (Gibson 2003, 5). To make his point absolutely clear, he states, "An adult who is born deaf who only learns sign is likely to be on a disability pension during their lifetime" (Gibson 2003, 9). And he stresses that their language is somewhat lacking, too: "It [Auslan] is a valid language although it lacks the grammatical structure of spoken and written English" (Gibson 1991, 213).

Such a depressing parade of inaccurate and fatuous comments about Deaf people suggests that very few health professionals who give advice to parents have any real knowledge of the Deaf community, its language, and its culture. How many have any real interest in acquiring this knowledge? We contend exceedingly few. Some in the medical profession do now pay lip service to the Deaf community and to Auslan because of the positive exposure the media has given Deaf people in recent years.

Commentators also misrepresent information by saying that deaf children (those who sign, the implication being deaf children without a cochlear implant) leave school with an average reading age of nine years. At face value, this information is not inaccurate; the statistic "average reading age of nine years" is commonly quoted by professionals and advocates of all persuasions. However, these commentators do not reveal that this reading age of nine is a result of lack of access to Auslan and education through Auslan. It is most common among deaf people who have been through an oral system—the system that rejects Auslan. Deaf children routinely are taught by teachers who do not use the language that is natural for the children use.

In other words, whose fault is it that deaf children are poorly educated? The education system? Or the fact of deafness? We would not tolerate a teacher of Vietnamese children who did not know the Vietnamese language.

DISPUTING THE CHESTNUTS

It might be good sport to pick off the occasional comments made by the medical profession and the captains of industry. What is more difficult is to counteract the persistent and patronizing chestnuts that are recycled year after year, particularly with parents who have discovered their child is deaf and who are confronting it. Here is our list of stale perspectives.

- *What we have heard:* "Signing interferes with learning speech" or "Signing makes them lazy and not want to bother to learn to speak."
  - *What we know from experience:* The assumption that Deaf people are lazy is patronizing. Deaf people have always had a range of abilities to speak, and this diversity will continue to be so. Nothing has changed.
- *What we have heard:* "Parents need to choose between speech and signing as well as between the Deaf community and the hearing community."
  - *What we know from experience:* Every Deaf person we know mixes with both. Numerous Deaf people have relationships with hearing people.
- *What we have heard:* "If hearing parents let their deaf child have access to the Deaf community, they will lose that child to the Deaf community."
  - *What we know from experience:* Ironically, parents who follow this thinking express a form of conditional love, saying to the child, "I will love you only if you do this, this, and this. Accepting any deaf child involves accepting that child's deafness as a part of who he or she is. A child whose deafness is accepted will never be lost to the parents.
- *What we have heard:* "If they must sign, signed English is better than Auslan."
  - *What we know from experience:* No one in the Deaf community knows or uses signed English.
- *What we have heard:* "The Deaf community will not accept deaf children who have a cochlear implant."
  - *What we know from experience:* Young Deaf people with cochlear implants are a normal and unremarkable sight at gatherings of the Deaf community.
- *What we have heard:* "Signing is a fallback, a last resort."
  - *What we know from experience:* Signing is an excellent medium in a world that is extremely noisy.

- *What we have heard:* "If they sign, their options will be limited; after all, not many people sign."
  - *What we know from experience:* Auslan is a language, and those fluent in it gain all the advantages of language. Evidence from Deaf societies suggests large numbers of hearing people are learning to sign or have some knowledge. Antidiscrimination legislation, the emergence of the profession of interpreting, and the value of diversity is opening up more opportunities for Deaf people.
- *What we have heard* (our favorite, and in our view the most ubiquitous of all, and deserving of the longest reply): "We all live in a hearing world" (WALIAHW).
  - *What we know from experience:* The "we all live in a hearing world" statement is the Deaf community's equivalent of the hearing statement, "live in the real world!" There is no such thing as a hearing world. As an expression, it is so vague as to be meaningless; therefore, it means anything anybody wants it to mean. Those who perceive deafness as a negative use WALIAHW to suggest that hearing people are important and Deaf people are insignificant. However, in its vagueness, it carries the same import as to say we all live in a world where the grass is green or where the sky is blue.

    We all associate with people who are like us. Everyone collects in their own little worlds, for example, retired conservative politicians, medical specialists, audiologists, journalists, computer nerds, film buffs, football fanatics, yachting enthusiasts, ethnic groups—any group of people who share common values and a sense of the world at large. Few people would attempt to describe the larger world to such enthusiasts through inverse terms, as for example, to say to yachties, "We all live in a world where most people are not interested in yachts."

Karen: During lunch one day at the parent conference I mentioned above, I sat across the table from a cochlear implant surgeon. He responded to some of my comments in my presentation. He insisted that the cochlear implant is good for children and that they do work with deaf adults. I later discovered his clinic works with a program for oral deaf adults, not Deaf people who sign.

During our conversation I said to him, "If you can tell me that kids with a cochlear implant have age-appropriate language—language, not speech—any language, Auslan or English, I don't care which, by the time they go to school, then I will say the cochlear implant is successful." And he replied, "Oh, but they do!"

"Age-appropriate language? All of them?" I asked incredulously.

"Yes, yes!" he insisted.

Now, I know his claim is not true for the majority of deaf children. In fact, I have yet to meet an implanted person for whom this claim is true. The only charitable conclusion I can make from this conversation is that his idea of "age-appropriate language" is vastly different from mine. Seeing firsthand a respected member of the medical profession insisting on stating information to me that I know is blatantly incorrect is mind boggling. But these are the people that parents and the media listen to and believe.

The Fallacies Go beyond Deaf People

Michael: My experience with parents of children with disabilities has been good and bad. The worst of these parents I encountered assumed a comprehensive knowledge of all disability based on their knowledge of their particular child. They treated me and others as overgrown children who needed a firm guiding hand. The best parents of children with disabilities were respectful; they listened, and they treated me and others as equals.

One's attitudes toward a child with a disability influence how one treats other people. Perhaps in other circumstances, say, outside the issues of disability and parents, I would have found the worst among those people obnoxious anyway. My earlier poor experiences with some of those parents were alleviated when I, too, became a parent. But I held fast to my sense of having been unjustly treated; my becoming a parent did not give those people a rosy tint.

My more recent experience in the area of disability suggests that we are now seeing the same signs as what has happened within the Deaf community—the emergence of some form of a disability culture. Just like those in the Deaf community, there are people with disabilities who are not interested in a cure. People with physical disabilities who have this mindset can be confronting to people without disabilities. The late Elizabeth Hastings, Australia's former disability discrimination commissioner, made an interesting comment:

> The Disability Discrimination Act is predicated on this fundamental assumption that disability is part of the human community, that people with disabilities are not different or separate from our community, but are an integral, belonging part of the whole. Certainly disability is not always convenient, attractive or desirable, but it is an ordinary attribute of being human.
>
> Even though my disability is also not especially convenient, attractive or desirable, it is my life and I have absolutely no wish for it to be otherwise. Not everybody will feel the same way about his or her circumstances. However many people with disabilities do think and feel the way I do—that we do not wish to be altered, cured or transformed. We do wish our equipment would work reliably, and that education, transport, shopping and professional and other services, work, entertainment, banking, insurance and information were accessible to us. (Hastings 1997)

Change the System, Not the Person

Antidiscrimination legislation, championed by disability pioneers such as Elizabeth Hastings, is entrenched in Australia at state and federal levels. It is a significant development for Deaf people.

The cochlear implant represents a surgical solution. It uses surgery to alter the child to suit a system of social organization that expects its participants to hear.

In contrast, equal opportunity legislation and a language policy that recognizes the bona fides of Auslan and the Deaf community work in the opposite direction to surgical intervention. Those approaches look first at what the person needs to gain equality of opportunity and then directs that the system be altered to meet those needs. Equal opportunity accepts diversity and difference as "normal" and as something to be adjusted to by the wider, largely privileged community.

Consider the example of captions in cinemas. The cochlear implant would, in theory, use surgery to alter the individual to meet the social norm that people should hear the soundtrack of a film. Antidiscrimination legislation, however, accepts that there are some people who do not hear and therefore directs alterations to the system to ensure that such people have the same opportunity as others to follow the soundtrack of a film.

Let's Eliminate Black People

In the name of the cochlear implant, some appalling statements have been made against Deaf people. If we accept the argument that the Deaf community forms a distinctive linguistic minority and that the features of this minority group have more in common with ethnicity than with disability, then we can revisit some earlier quotes and look at their effect by changing some key words. So let us therefore substitute *Whites* for *hearing people*, *Black* for *Deaf*, and *Whitening Pill* for *cochlear implant*.

Now we see that in 1987 when Dr. Terry Hambrecht announced a major funding grant for the cochlear implant research program, he could have been saying in effect, "The goal of the research is to eliminate blackness, in the way diseases such as smallpox had been controlled." And former Liberal MHR Peter Howson could have been saying, "It may well be that in forty years time there will not be a Black community today as we know it." And Jack O'Mahoney could have been saying in effect, "Black people are a burden, but our Whitening Pill turns them into taxpayers and productive members of society." And Professor Bill Gibson could have been saying, "All Black people are under employed or unemployed and end up on a disability pension," and "The language used by Black people has no grammatical structure."

THE REALITY OF TODAY

Karen: In about 1997, when I was on the Board of AAD, we were at a strategic planning retreat and the cochlear implant was being discussed in terms of its effect on the deaf community and what AAD should be doing. Robert Adam (who is from a Deaf family) said he didn't think we needed to be so concerned about it. He said that the situation would develop just as it had with hearing aids and oralism, that kids with cochlear implants would go through oral programs and leave school and then come knocking on the door of the Deaf community, looking for themselves. We would open up the door and say, oh alright, come in, and then we would proceed to "fix them up," undo the damage as best we could, just as the Deaf community has done for generations of Deaf youths with hearing aids and an oral upbringing. Robert predicted that the Deaf community would simply absorb those with the cochlear implant and carry on. His prediction is what we are seeing now.

Now, some twenty years after the cochlear implant first began to cause consternation, maybe we are all settling down. The old divisions between those with and without a cochlear implant are becoming blurred. The situation is similar to the introduction of hearing aids and to the earlier groups of deaf people who were raised under the oral system.

Michael: In the end, the Deaflympics, held in Melbourne in January 2005, provided the best possible response to the cochlear implant by the world Deaf community—a profound lack of interest. There were athletes and officials with cochlear implants, and no one noticed or cared. During the games, I caught up with many people. Some had hearing aids, some had a cochlear implant, some had neither. I talked to some, I signed to others, and with one or two I got by with a hybrid version of American fingerspelling and International Sign. The Deaflympics indicated that cochlear implants have arrived, just as hearing aids did a generation or two ago. The Deaf community flexed and adjusted to Deaf people with hearing aids, just as it is doing now for those with the cochlear implant. There at the games was when I understood: the effect of banal arrogance has gone. It is now just a cliché, a brief sputtering outrage that surfaced briefly. It is not, and never was, the cochlear implant itself that was so damaging. It was the way hearing people used it to demonize Deaf people.

David Wright, the poet whose observation we introduced at the beginning of this chapter, died in 1994 at the age of 74. His obituary in the Melbourne newspaper *The Age* (1994) had this to say:

Internationally acclaimed South African-born poet David Wright did not believe being deaf since childhood had been much of a handicap. Rather, the affliction had been a "stimulus" for him to see the world in a different way to others. He once said in an interview "I do not notice more but I notice differently. . . . [T]he deaf person watches from the unexpected and unguarded quarter."

David Wright inadvertently spelled out the greatest fear of hearing professionals to Deaf people: that these clients, these helpless burdens on society, these underemployed, unfulfilled, language-deprived, and suffering deaf who are doomed to a world of silence and who survive on disability pensions, may know far more than they let on.

Deaf people in Australia, and around the world, have endured because of the simplest of reasons: other Deaf people are the people with whom they can communicate most easily. The same applies to hard of hearing people and explains why, despite their allegiance to the "hearing world," they do congregate in groups like Better Hearing Australia and Self Help for the Hard of Hearing. No medical technology will change the profound ease of communication among Deaf people, among those who are hard of hearing, and among those with the cochlear implant who flock to both groups.

Notes

1. Passages indicated by "Karen" and "Michael" represent commentary by the authors of this chapter.
2. "The kingdom of speech . . . is a realm whose queen tolerates no rivals. Speech is jealous and wishes to be absolute mistress" (Reverend Giulio Tarra, peroration at 1880 Congress of Milan cited in Lane 1984, 393).
3. VCOD's (Victorian Council of Deaf People) forum on the cochlear implant in August 1988 featured hearing and Deaf parents, a Deaf teacher, an adult cochlear implant recipient, and an audiologist from the cochlear implant program. We understand that, more recently, Professor Graeme Clark has spoken at Deaf functions in Melbourne.

References

Ackehurst, S. 2000. *Broken silence,* Sydney: Harper Collins, Allen & Unwin.

The Age. 1994. David Wright (obituary), September 8.

Clark, G. 2000. *Sounds from Silence.* Sydney, Australia: Allen & Unwin.

Gibson, W. 1991. Opposition from deaf groups to the CI. *Medical Journal of Australia* 155 (19):213.

———. 2003. Understanding hearing loss—Part I. *Hearing Matters* (publication of Australia's Self Help for Hard of Hearing) (February).

Haenke, M. 1988. Letters to the editor. *SHHH News,* May 11.

Hastings, E. 1997. Keynote address. Presented at the Social Options Conference, November 21, Adelaide, Australia.

Komesaroff, L. 2003. Allegations of unlawful discrimination in education: Parents taking their fight for Auslan to courts. *Journal of Deaf Studies and Deaf Education* 9: 210–80.

Lane, H. 1984. *When the mind hears: A history of the deaf.* New York: Random House.

Lo Bianco, J. 1987. *National policy on languages.* Canberra: Government Printer.

Menagh, C. 1987. United States backs study to perfect a bionic ear. *The Age* (Melbourne), March 5, 1.

Pheasant, B. 2003. The band leader. *AFR Boss,* August 9.

Stephens, T. 1994. The world watches Sally switch on her ears. *Sydney Morning Herald,* December 3, 3.

Uniacke, M. 1987. Of miracles, praise—and anger—the bionic ear. *Future, Commission for the Future* 6 (August): 11–14.

Wright, D. 1969. *Deafness.* New York: Stein and Day.

INDEX